Applied Econometrics for Health Economists

A practical guide

Second Edition

Andrew Jones
Professor of Economics
Department of Economics and Related Studies
University of York

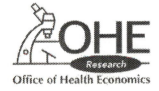

Office of Health Economics

Radcliffe Publishing
Oxford • Seattle

Radcliffe Publishing Ltd
18 Marcham Road
Abingdon
Oxon OX14 1AA
United Kingdom

www.radcliffe-oxford.com
Electronic catalogue and worldwide online ordering facility.

British Library Cataloguing in Publication Data

A catalogue record for this book is available from the British Library.

ISBN-10: 1 84619 171 8
ISBN-13: 978 1 84619 171 8

Typeset by Lapiz Digital Services, Chennai, India
Printed and bound by Biddles Ltd, King's Lynn, Norfolk, UK

Contents

Preface

Given the extensive use of individual-level survey data in health economics, it is important to understand the econometric techniques available to applied researchers. Moreover, it is just as important to be aware of their limitations and pitfalls. The purpose of this book is to introduce readers to the appropriate econometric techniques for use with different forms of survey data – known collectively as microeconometrics. There is a strong emphasis on applied work, illustrating the use of relevant computer software applied to large-scale survey data sets. The aim is to illustrate the steps involved in doing microeconometric research:

- formulate empirical problems involving large survey data sets
- construct usable data sets and know the limitations of survey design
- select an appropriate econometric method
- be aware of the methods of estimation that are available for microeconometric models and the software that can be used to implement them
- interpret the results of the analysis and describe their implications in a statistically and economically meaningful way.

The standard linear regression model, familiar from econometric textbooks, is designed to deal with a dependent variable that varies continuously over a range between minus infinity and plus infinity. Unfortunately, this standard model is rarely applicable with survey data, where qualitative and categorical variables are more common. This book therefore deals with practical analysis of qualitative and categorical variables. The book assumes basic familiarity with the principles of statistical inference – estimation and hypothesis testing – and with the linear regression model. An accessible and clear overview of the linear regression model is given in the fifth edition of Peter Kennedy's book *A Guide to Econometrics*, published by MIT Press, and the material is covered in many other introductory econometrics textbooks.

Technical details or derivations are avoided in the main text and the book concentrates on the intuition behind the models and their interpretation. Key terms are marked in **bold** and defined in the Glossary. Formulae and more technical details are presented in the Technical appendix; the structure of the appendix follows that of the main text, with the numbered sections in the appendix corresponding to the chapters in the main text. References are kept to a minimum to maintain the flow of the text and are augmented with a list of further Recommended reading for readers who would like to pursue the topics in more detail. All of the results presented are estimated using Stata (www.stata.com/). Examples of relevant Stata commands are described and explained in an appendix to each chapter, and a separate Software appendix lists the full set of Stata commands that can be used to compute the methods and empirical examples used in the text. To give a feel for the way that the software package presents results, the tables are reproduced as they appear in the Stata output. The text refers to key results only and readers who want a full explanation of all of the statistics listed are encouraged to consult the Stata user manuals.

Andrew Jones
November 2006

About the author

Andrew Jones is professor of economics at the University of York, where he directs the graduate programme in health economics, and visiting professor at the University of Bergen. He is research director of the Health, Econometrics and Data Group (HEDG) at the University of York. He researches and publishes extensively in the area of microeconometrics and health economics. He is an organiser of the European Workshops on Econometrics and Health Economics and coordinator of the Marie Curie Training Programme in Applied Health Economics. He has edited the *Elgar Companion to Health Economics*, is joint editor of *Health Economics* and of *Health Economics Letters*, and is an associate editor of the *Journal of Health Economics*.

Acknowledgements

I am grateful to my colleagues in the Health, Econometrics and Data Group (HEDG) at the University of York for their helpful comments and suggestions on earlier versions of the book, and to Hugh Gravelle, Carol Propper and Frank Windmeijer for their insightful and comprehensive reviews of the material. Thanks to Jon Sussex, who provided me with the original challenge of preparing a non-technical guide to econometrics for health economists, 'without equations'.

Chapter 1

Introduction: the evaluation problem and linear regression

The evaluation problem

The evaluation problem is how to identify causal effects from empirical data. An understanding of the implications of the evaluation problem for statistical analysis will help to provide a motivation for many of the econometric methods discussed below.

Consider an outcome y_{it}, for individual i at time t; for example an individual's level of use of healthcare services over the past year. The problem is to identify the effect of a treatment, for example whether the individual has purchased private health insurance, on the outcome. The causal effect of interest is the difference between the outcome with the treatment and the outcome without the treatment. But this pure treatment effect cannot be identified from empirical data. This is because the counterfactual can never be observed. The basic problem is that the individual 'cannot be in two places at the same time'; that is, we cannot observe their use of healthcare at time t, both with and without the influence of insurance.

One response to this problem is to concentrate on the **average treatment effect** and attempt to estimate it with sample data by comparing the average outcome among those receiving the treatment with the average outcome among those who do not receive the treatment. The problem for statistical inference arises if there are unobserved factors that influence both whether an individual is selected into the treatment group and also how they respond to the treatment. This will lead to biased estimates of the treatment effect. For example, someone who knows they have a high risk of illness may be more prone to take out health insurance and they will also tend to use more healthcare. Unless the analyst is able to control for their level of risk, this will lead to spurious evidence of a positive relationship between having health insurance and using healthcare.

A randomised experimental design – which randomises the allocation of individuals into treatments – may be able to control for this bias and, in some circumstances, a natural experiment may mimic the features of a controlled experiment. However, the vast majority of econometric studies rely on observational data gathered in a non-experimental setting. In the absence of experimental data, attention has to focus on alternative estimation strategies.

- **Instrumental variables (IV)**: variables (or 'instruments') that are good predictors of the treatment, but are not independently related to the outcome, may be used to purge the bias. In practice, the validity of the IV approach relies on finding appropriate instruments and these may be hard to find (*see* Jones 2000 and Auld 2006 for further discussion).
- Corrections for selection bias: these range from parametric methods such as the **Heckit** estimator to more recent semiparametric estimators. The use of these techniques in health economics is discussed in Chapter 7.

- Longitudinal data: the availability of **panel data**, giving repeated measurements for a particular individual, provides the opportunity to control for unobservable individual effects which remain constant over time. Panel data models are discussed in Chapter 11.

Classical linear regression

So far, the discussion has concentrated on the evaluation problem. More generally, most econometric work in health economics focuses on the problem of finding an appropriate model to fit the available data. Classical linear regression analysis assumes that the relationship between an outcome, or dependent variable, y, and the explanatory variables or independent variables, x, can be summarised by a regression function. The regression function is typically assumed to be a linear function of the x variables and of a random error term, ε. This relationship can be written using the following shorthand notation:

$$y = x\beta + \varepsilon. \tag{1}$$

The random error term ε captures all of the variation in y that is not explained by the x variables. The classical model assumes that:

- this error term has a mean of zero
- that its variance, σ^2, is the same across all the observations (this is known as **homoskedasticity**)
- that values of the error term are independent across observations (known as **serial independence**)
- that values of the error term are independent of the values of the x variables (known as **exogeneity**).

Often it is assumed that the error term has a **normal distribution**. This implies that, conditional on each observation's x_i, each observation of the dependent variable y_i should follow a normal distribution with mean equal to $x_i\beta$.

So far we have not specified how y is measured. Often the quantity that is of direct economic interest will be transformed before it is entered into the regression model. For example, data on household healthcare expenditures or on the costs of an episode of treatment have non-negative values only and tend to have highly skewed distributions, with many small values and a long right-hand tail with a few exceptionally expensive cases. Regression analyses of these kinds of skewed data often transform the raw scale, for example by taking logarithms, before running the regression analysis. This reduces the skewness of the distribution and makes the assumption of normality more reasonable. However, the economic interpretation of the results is usually carried out on the original scale, in units of expenditure, and care needs to be taken in retransforming back to this scale. This is particularly true in the presence of **heteroskedasticity**. There is an extensive literature in health economics on this **retransformation problem**, which explores the properties of the logarithmic and other related transformations (*see*, for example, Manning 2006).

In health economics, empirical analysis is complicated by the fact that the theoretical models often involve inherently unobservable (latent) concepts such as health endowments, physician agency and supplier inducement, or quality of life. The widespread use of individual-level survey data means that nonlinear models are common in health economics, as measures of outcomes are often based on qualitative or limited dependent variables. Examples of these nonlinear models include:

- binary responses, such as whether the individual has visited their GP over the previous month (*see* Chapter 3)
- multinomial responses, such as the choice of healthcare provider (*see* Chapters 4 and 5)
- integer counts, such as the number of GP visits (*see* Chapter 9)
- measures of duration, such as the time elapsed between visits (*see* Chapter 10).

Throughout the rest of the book, emphasis is placed on the assumptions underpinning these econometric models and applied empirical examples are provided. The empirical examples are based on a single data set, the Health and Lifestyle Survey of Great Britain (HALS). The next chapter describes how the survey was collected and the kind of information it contains.

Chapter 2

The Health and Lifestyle Survey

Survey design

The Health and Lifestyle Survey (HALS) was designed as a representative survey of adults in Great Britain (*see* Cox *et al.* 1987, 1993). The population surveyed was individuals aged 18 and over living in private households. In principle, each individual should have an equal probability of being selected for the survey. This allows the data to be used to make inferences about the underlying population. HALS was designed originally as a **cross-section survey** with one measurement for each observation, or individual. It was carried out between the autumn of 1984 and the summer of 1985. Information was collected in three stages:

- a one-hour face-to-face interview, which collected information on experience and attitudes towards to health and lifestyle along with general socioeconomic information
- a nurse visit to collect physiological measures and indicators of cognitive function, such as memory and reasoning
- a self-completion postal questionnaire to measure psychiatric health and personality.

The HALS is an example of a clustered random sample. The intention was to build a representative random sample of this population. Addresses were randomly selected from electoral registers using a three-stage design. First, 198 electoral constituencies were selected with the probability of selection proportional to the population of each constituency. Then two wards were selected for each constituency and, finally, 30 addresses per ward. Individuals were randomly selected from households. This selection procedure gave a target of 12,672 interviews.

Some of the addresses from the electoral register proved to be inappropriate as they were in use as holiday homes, business premises or were derelict (*see* Table 2.1 for details). This number was relatively small, and only 418 addresses were excluded, leaving a total of 12,254 individuals to be interviewed. The response rate fell more dramatically when it came to success in completing these interviews. A total of 9,003 interviews were completed (*see* Table 2.2). This is a response rate of 73.5%. In other words, there was a roughly 1 in 4 chance that an interview was not completed. The missing values are an example of **unit non-response**. For these individuals, no information is available from any of the survey questions. The main reason for non-response is refusal on the part of the interviewee or their family. This accounted for 2,341 cases or 19% of the requests for interview. Further cases were lost because the interviewer was unable to establish contact or for other reasons, such as illness or incapacity on the part of the interviewee.

A question for researchers is whether the 1 in 4 individuals who were not included in the survey are systematically different from those who did respond. If there are systematic differences, this creates a problem of **sample selection bias** and it will not be possible to claim that inferences based on the observed data are representative of the underlying population (*see* Chapter 7). What do we know

Table 2.1: Selection of addresses for HALS

	Number	*%*
Addresses selected	12,672	100
Reasons for exclusion		
Vacant/holiday home/derelict	338	
Business	15	
Demolished	14	
No private household	12	
No one aged 18+	1	
Untraced	38	
Total exclusions	418	3.3
Total included	12,254	96.7

Table 2.2: Response to requests for interviews in HALS

	Number	*%*
Total requests	12,254	100
Reasons for not interviewing		
Refusal (personal or other household member)	2,341	19.1
Failure to establish contact	646	5.3
Other reasons (senile or incapacitated, too ill, inadequate English, etc.)	264	2.2
Interviews achieved	9,003	73.5

about the people who did not participate in the interview? Although the survey provides no information, we do know the addresses of the non-responders. This allows us to compare response rates across geographic areas and to use other sources of information about those areas (*see* Table 2.3). For example, analysis of the HALS data shows that response rates were particularly low in Greater London, with a response rate of 64.2% compared to 73.5% on average. The representativeness of the sample can be gauged further by comparing the observed data to external data sources. So, for example, the HALS team compared their survey to the 1981 census (*see* Table 2.4). This comparison suggests that the HALS data under-represent men and over-represent women, with only 43.4% of men among the interviewees compared to 47.7% in the census population.

The overall response rate of 73.5% is fairly typical of general population surveys. Understandably, the response rate declines for the subsequent nurse visit and postal questionnaire. The overall response rate for those individuals who completed all three stages of the survey is only 53.7%. Comparison with the 1981 census suggests that this final sample under-represents those with lower incomes and lower levels of education. It is important to bear unit non-response in mind when doing any analysis with survey data sets.

A further source of missing data is **item non-response**. This occurs when an individual responds to the interview as a whole but is unwilling or unable to answer a particular question. Non-responses are coded as 'missing values' in the

Table 2.3: Response rates across regions in HALS

Interview	Population number	Achieved number	Achieved %
Scotland	1,160	925	79.7
Wales	626	500	79.9
North	681	542	79.6
North West	1,498	1,098	73.3
Yorkshire & Humberside	1,106	812	73.4
West Midlands	1,112	827	74.4
East Midlands	877	685	78.1
East Anglia	433	333	76.9
South West	987	721	73.0
South East	2,303	1,615	70.1
Greater London	1,471	945	64.2
Total	12,254	9,003	73.5

Table 2.4: Characteristics of HALS sample compared to 1981 Census

Age	Census	Int*	Nurse**	Post***	Census	Int	Nurse	Post
	% Men				% Women			
18–20	6.9	5.8	5.8	5.7	6.1	5.0	4.8	4.9
21–29	17.9	17.2	16.5	15.6	16.1	16.4	16.6	16.5
30–39	19.6	19.8	20.8	20.8	17.7	20.6	22.8	23.1
40–49	16.0	16.6	17.0	16.5	14.5	16.7	17.4	17.1
50–59	16.1	15.1	15.3	15.8	15.3	14.7	14.7	15.0
60–69	13.2	13.9	13.7	14.4	14.1	14.5	13.7	14.3
70+	10.2	11.6	10.9	11.1	16.2	12.0	10.1	9.2
All	47.7	43.4	44.8	44.3	52.3	56.6	55.2	55.7

* Interview; **Nurse visit; ***Postal questionnaire

data set. Again, researchers should be aware of the potential bias this creates if observations with missing values are systematically different from those who respond to the question. For example, the self-employed may be less willing to reveal information about their income than those in paid employment. Chapter 7 discusses some of the methods that can be used to deal with non-response and the sample selection bias it can create.

The longitudinal follow-up

The HALS data were originally intended to be a one-off cross-section survey and most of the examples used in this book are drawn from the original cross-section. However, HALS also provides an example of a longitudinal or **panel data** set. In 1991/92, seven years on from the original survey, the HALS was repeated. This provides an example of repeated measurements where the same individuals are re-interviewed. Panel data provide a powerful enhancement of cross-section surveys that allows a deeper analysis of heterogeneity across individuals and of changes in individual behaviour over time. However, because of the need to revisit and interview individuals repeatedly, the problems of **unit non-response** tend to be amplified. Of the original 9,003 individuals who were interviewed at the time of the first HALS survey, 808 (9%) had died by the time of the second survey, 1,347 (14.9%) could not be traced and 222 were traced but could not be interviewed, either because they had moved overseas or they had moved to geographic areas that were outside the scope of the survey. These cases are examples of attrition – individuals who drop out of a longitudinal survey. Systematic differences between the individuals who stay in and those who drop out can lead to **attrition bias**. This is discussed in more detail in Chapter 11.

The deaths data

HALS provides an example of a cross-section survey (HALS1) and panel data (HALS1&2). It also provides a longitudinal follow-up of subseqent mortality and cancer cases among the original respondents. These deaths data can be used for survival analysis (*see* Chapter 10). Most of the 9,003 individuals interviewed in HALS1, have been *flagged* on the NHS Central Register. In June 2005, the fifth death revision and the second cancer revision were completed. The flagging process was quite lengthy because it required several checks in order to be sure that the flagging registrations were related to the person previously interviewed. As reported in Table 2.5, about 98% of the sample has been flagged. Deaths account for some 27% of the original sample.

Table 2.5: Deaths data, June 2005 release

Status in June 2005 deaths data	Number of cases	%
On file	6,248	69.4
Not NHS register	85	0.94
Deceased	2,431	27.0
Reported dead, not identified	1	0.01
Embarked abroad	42	0.05
No flag yet received	196	2.18

Socioeconomic characteristics

Most of the empirical models shown in this book use a common set of individual socioeconomic characteristics as explanatory variables (also know as independent variables or regressors). These include examples of continuous variables, whose values can be treated as varying continuously (in practice these kinds of variables may include integer-valued variables that have sufficient variability to be treated as approximating a continuous variable). The example of a 'continuous' variable in our data is the individual's age (*age*), which is measured in years. To allow for a flexible relationship between age and the outcomes of interest, squared and cubic terms are included in the models as well (*age2* and *age3*). Also age is centred around age 45 (the reason for this is explained below). All of the other regressors are indicator variables (also know as **dummy variables**). These take a value of 1 if an individual has a particular characteristic and 0 otherwise. The dummy variables are included in groups. There is a single indicator for gender (*male*). Ethnic group is split into: black and West Indian; Indian, Pakistani and Bangladeshi; and other non-white (*ethbawi, ethipb, ethothnw*). Employment status covers part-time employed, unemployed, retired, full-time students and keeping house (*part, unemp, retd, stdnt, keephse*). Education is measured by the age that an individual left full-time education: under 14, 14, 15, 17, 18 or over 18 (*lsch14u, lsch14, lsch15, lsch17, lsch18, lsch19*). Social class is measured by the Registrar General's occupational social class (*regscls, regsc2, regsc3n, regsc4, regsc5n*). Marital status includes widowed, never married, separated and divorced (*widow, single, seprd, divorce*). It should be clear that each of these groups has an omitted category. This is to avoid the 'dummy variables trap' that would create perfect collinearity in the regression models if a dummy variable was included for every category. The omitted categories are female, white, employed, left school at 16, social class 3 manual and married; and the reference age is 45. Together these define the 'reference individual', a concept that is discussed in more detail below.

Table 2.6 shows descriptive statistics, produced using the 'summarise' command in Stata, for the full list of socioeconomic variables. These show that 43% of the sample are men and the average age is 46, with a range from 18 to 98. There are relatively few respondents from non-white ethnic minorities represented in the sample. After full-time employees (the omitted employment

Table 2.6: Descriptive statistics for the HALS data

Variable	Obs	Mean	Std. Dev.	Min	Max
male	9003	.4337443	.4956183	0	1
age	9003	46.44907	17.72568	18	98
ethbawi	9003	.010441	.1016518	0	1
ethipb	9003	.0143286	.1188479	0	1
ethothnw	9003	.0072198	.0846669	0	1
part	9003	.1210708	.3262276	0	1
unemp	9003	.0504276	.2188379	0	1
retd	9003	.221926	.4155647	0	1
stdnt	9003	.011996	.1088734	0	1
keephse	9003	.1401755	.3471883	0	1
lsch14u	9003	.0377652	.1906384	0	1
lsch14	9003	.2515828	.4339468	0	1
lsch15	9003	.2716872	.4448542	0	1
lsch17	9003	.0880818	.2834295	0	1
lsch18	9003	.088415	.2839132	0	1
lsch19	9003	.0133289	.1146852	0	1
regscls	9003	.0570921	.2320314	0	1
regsc2	9003	.2230368	.4163059	0	1
regsc3n	9003	.1405087	.3475334	0	1
regsc4	9003	.167944	.3738373	0	1
regsc5n	9003	.0607575	.2388983	0	1
widow	9003	.0865267	.2811559	0	1
single	9003	.1704987	.3760912	0	1
seprd	9003	.0219927	.1466676	0	1
divorce	9003	.0377652	.1906384	0	1

category), the retired are the next largest group, with 22% of the sample. Most commonly, respondents left school at age 16 (the omitted category), followed by 15 and 14. The majority are married (the omitted category), followed by those who had never married at the time of the survey.

Appendix: Stata code for data handling and descriptive statistics

The HALS data are stored as a Stata dataset. The first step is to load the Stata dataset into the package. This can be done with the 'use' command:

```
use 'c:\....\...\your_filename.dta', clear
```

It is helpful to open a log file that will store a permanent record of the output of the session:

```
log using 'c:\...\...\your_filename.log', replace
```

Considerable time and effort can be saved by creating a 'global' for the list of variable names. This avoids having to type them out in full in subsequent commands. Here a global 'xvars' is created that lists all of the socioeconomic variables that will be used in the regression models:

```
global xvars 'male age age2 age3 ethbawi ethipb ethothnw
part unemp retd stdnt keephse
lsch14u lsch14 lsch15 lsch17 lsch18 lsch19
regsc1s regsc2 regsc3n regsc4 regsc5n
widow single seprd divorce
partime retired student keephouse'
```

This global can then be used in the 'summarise' command to provide descriptive statistics for the variables:

```
summ $xvars
```

One way of assessing the importance of non-response is to compare the descriptive statistics for the sample of observations that are used to estimate the regression model and the sample of available observations that are not used. Here a regression model for self-assessed health (sah) is used to create an indicator variable for those observations that are selected into the sample. A convenient feature of Stata is 'e(sample)', an indicator of whether or not an observation was in the sample used to estimate the regression model. This is used to create the indicator 'miss', so that the descriptive statistics can be calculated separately 'by' the values of miss (i.e. for the estimation sample and for the remaining sample):

```
gen yvar = sah
quietly regr yvar $xvars
gen miss=0
recode miss 0=1 if e(sample)
sort miss
by miss: summ $xvars
```

Chapter 3

Binary dependent variables

Methods

It is often the case in survey data that the outcome of interest is measured as a **binary variable**, taking values of either one or zero. Often this binary variable will indicate whether an individual is a participant or a non-participant. Examples include: healthcare utilisation, such as whether an individual has visited a GP in the previous month; or whether they have used prescription drugs; or whether a household has purchased health insurance; or whether an individual is a current smoker. If the binary outcome y, depends on a set of explanatory variables x, then the conditional expectation of y given x, in other words the value of y that individuals with characteristics x are likely to report on average, is:

$$E(y|x) = 0.P(y = 0|x) + 1.P(y = 1|x) = P(y = 1|x) = F(x). \quad (2)$$

A simple way to model binary data is to use a linear function, for which we can use the shorthand notation, $F(x) = x\beta$. This gives the **linear probability model**, which is straightforward to estimate, using standard software for the method of **ordinary least squares**.

These estimates should be adjusted for the fact that, by design, the error term in the equation cannot have a normal distribution. Normality implies that the error is continuous and can take any value between plus and minus infinity. In the linear probability model, the error term can take only two values corresponding to values of zero or one for the dependent variable. The variance of this implied error term depends on the x-values. In other words, by design, the error term is **heteroskedastic** (meaning that its variance differs across individuals with different values of x). This can be corrected by using a **robust estimator** of the standard errors, while using **weighted least squares** rather than ordinary least squares can improve the efficiency of the estimates.

In practice, the linear probability model may provide a reasonable approximation for binary choice models, so long as the function F(.) is approximately linear over the range of sample observations. But a major drawback of the method is that, because a straight line is used, predicted values of the regression function can lie outside the range zero to one. Equation (2) shows that these predicted values correspond to the probability that an individual participates. This means that the linear probability model can lead to logical inconsistencies, with predicted probabilities outside the logical range zero to one. A way to avoid this is to use a non-linear function for F(.). Popular choices are 'S' curves, which are bounded to the range [0,1] whatever the values of the regressors x. The most common choices of these 'S' curves are **logit** and **probit** models.

Logit and probit models are often motivated in terms of a latent variable specification. This assumes that there is some continuous latent variable y* that determines participation. You can think of y* as an individual's propensity to participate. If y* is positive, the individual will choose to participate and the observed binary outcome equals 1. Otherwise, the individual will not participate and the observed value equals 0. Then the latent variable y* is modelled by a linear regression function of the individual characteristics x. Assuming that the error term in this equation has a standard normal distribution gives the probit model. Assuming that it has a standard **logistic distribution** gives the logit model. The probability functions for the probit and logit models both have the characteristic 'S' shape and are similar in appearance, although the logit model gives more weight to the tails of the distribution. As with many of the models described in this book, logit and probit models are typically estimated by the method of **maximum likelihood estimation**. This method is discussed in more detail in the technical appendix.

Results for the linear probability model

To illustrate the estimation and interpretation of linear probability, logit and probit models, we will use HALS data on individuals' self-assessed health. In HALS, self-assessed health is measured on a four-point scale, with categories 'excellent', 'good', 'fair' and 'poor'. To illustrate binary choice models, this is collapsed into a binary variable where y = 1, if an individual reports excellent or good health, and y = 0, if an individual reports fair or poor health. The aim is to model the probability of an individual reporting excellent or good health as a function of a range of socioeconomic characteristics, including the individual's gender, age, ethnic origin, work status, educational qualifications, occupational socioeconomic group and marital status.

Table 3.1 presents the **weighted least squares (WLS)** estimates for the linear probability model. These are computed in two steps. First, the model is estimated using **ordinary least squares (OLS)** and the predicted values from this equation are saved. These predictions are then used to calculate weights. This is possible only if the predictions lie within the range [0,1]. So, any logically inconsistent predictions mean that it is not possible to use weighted least squares. In the example reported here, this was not a problem as all of the predictions are in the required range.

One attraction of the linear probability model is its ease of interpretation. As we have seen in equation (2), the regression function, E(y|x), can be interpreted as the probability of participating given the values of x, and here this is assumed to be a linear function. This means that the regression coefficients β are measured in units of probability. So, for example consider the constant term 0.754 (in the final row of Table 3.1). This is the value of the regression function when all of the x variables equal 0. You can think of this as a 'reference individual'. In this example, the x variables have been constructed so that the reference individual is a woman aged 45 who is white, in full-time employment, left school at 16, is in a skilled manual occupation and is married. The coefficient tells us that this type of individual has a probability of 0.754 of reporting excellent or good health, rather than fair or poor health.

The coefficients on the x variables tell us how this probability changes with changes in the individual's characteristics. The regression function includes two types of explanatory variable. The first type can be treated as though they were **continuous variables**. The example here is the individual's age measured in

Table 3.1: Linear probability model of sah (WLS)

Source	SS	df	MS	
				Number of obs = 8895
				F(27, 8867) = 13.02
Model	71.8679703	27	2.66177668	Prob > F = 0.0000
Residual	1813.16391	8867	.204484483	R-squared = 0.0381
				Adj R-squared = 0.0352
Total	1885.03188	8894	.211944219	Root MSE = .4522

yvar	Coef.	Std. Err.	t	P>|t|	[95% Conf. Interval]	
male	.0110496	.0116204	0.95	0.342	−.0117291	.0338283
age	−.0028952	.0007957	−3.64	0.000	−.0044549	−.0013354
age2	−.0107486	.0028589	−3.76	0.000	−.0163527	−.0051444
age3	.0404218	.0095455	4.23	0.000	.0217105	.0591331
ethbawi	−.1076602	.0435029	−2.47	0.013	−.1929359	−.0223845
ethipb	−.0876126	.038631	−2.27	0.023	−.1633383	−.0118869
ethothnw	−.1256814	.0542635	−2.32	0.021	−.2320504	−.0193124
part	.0644476	.018349	3.51	0.000	.0284793	.100416
unemp	−.0445345	.021623	−2.06	0.039	−.0869206	−.0021485
retd	.0193786	.0209592	0.92	0.355	−.0217062	.0604634
stdnt	.072331	.0536686	1.35	0.178	−.0328719	.177534
keephse	−.0292059	.0168368	−1.73	0.083	−.0622098	.003798
lsch14u	−.0743648	.0281281	−2.64	0.008	−.1295023	−.0192273
lsch14	−.075411	.0178249	−4.23	0.000	−.1103518	−.0404701
lsch15	−.0407599	.0147827	−2.76	0.006	−.0697375	−.0117823
lsch17	.0146558	.020515	0.71	0.475	−.0255583	.05487
lsch18	.0798895	.0233398	3.42	0.001	.0341381	.1256409
lsch19	.0114685	.0454503	0.25	0.801	−.0776246	.1005616
regsc1s	.0966774	.0272621	3.55	0.000	.0432373	.1501174
regsc2	.0772081	.0144526	5.34	0.000	.0488776	.1055385
regsc3n	.0351518	.0155857	2.26	0.024	.0046003	.0657033
regsc4	−.0281103	.0135481	−2.07	0.038	−.0546678	−.0015528
regsc5n	−.0674235	.0195772	−3.44	0.001	−.1057993	−.0290476
widow	−.0556353	.0185643	−3.00	0.003	−.0920257	−.0192449
single	−.0309911	.0166773	−1.86	0.063	−.0636824	.0017002
seprd	−.097271	.0311903	−3.12	0.002	−.1584112	−.0361309
divorce	−.0648466	.0243986	−2.66	0.008	−.1126735	−.0170196
_cons	.7544911	.0179991	41.92	0.000	.7192087	.7897735

RESET test;
   F(1, 8866) = 4.42
   Prob > F = 0.0355

years. All of the other explanatory variables are **binary** or **dummy variables**. These take the value 1 if the individual has a particular characteristic, for example if they are unemployed, and 0 otherwise.

An important general tool for interpreting the impact of changes in the regressors on the probability of participation is the **partial effect**. The way of calculating the partial effect depends on whether the regressor is continuous or discrete. For continuous explanatory variables, we look at the impact of a small change in the variable on the probability of participation. This is known as the

marginal effect. Here we could look at the impact of age on the probability of reporting excellent or good health. For the dummy variables, it does not make sense to think in terms of small changes. An individual either has a characteristic or does not. Here, we look at the **average effect**, for example the difference in the probability of reporting excellent or good health if someone is unemployed compared to someone who is employed.

An attraction of the linear probability model is that the regression coefficients measure directly both the marginal effect of continuous explanatory variables and the average effect of dummy explanatory variables.

The *sign* of the coefficients tells us about the **qualitative effect** of the explanatory variables. For example, Table 3.1 shows that the coefficient on unemployment is negative (−0.045). This means that an individual who is currently unemployed has a lower probability of reporting good or excellent health relative to the reference individual who is employed. The size of the coefficient tells us about the **quantitative effect** of the variable. The coefficient on unemployment is −0.045. This is measured in units of probability and tells us that the probability of reporting good or excellent health is 0.045 lower for someone who is unemployed than for the reference individual.

We are relying on a **point estimate** (−0.045) of the impact of unemployment. The fact that this estimate is different from zero may simply be due to chance, attributable to sampling variability. This sampling variability is summarised by the standard error of the coefficient. The null hypothesis that the coefficient equals zero can be tested by looking at the t-ratio, given by the ratio of the coefficient to its standard error. The t-ratios are reported in the fourth column of Table 3.1 and the corresponding p-value (the implied significance level of the test) is given in the fifth column. With a t-ratio of −2.06, we can say that the coefficient on unemployment is statistically significant at a conventional 5% level of significance ($p = 0.039$).

Now consider the other variables included in the model. The qualitative effects for occupational socioeconomic group show that those in social classes 1, 2 and 3 (non-manual) have positive coefficients. In other words, they are more likely to report good or excellent health compared to the reference individual who is in social class 3 – skilled manual occupations. Individuals in social classes 4 and 5 – semi-skilled and unskilled occupations – have negative coefficients, showing that, on average, they are less likely to report good or excellent health. The quantitative effects show some evidence of a gradient in health across socioeconomic groups.

A similar pattern emerges for education. Here, the reference category is leaving school at age 16. The qualitative effects show that those who left school at 15, 14 or under are less likely to report good or excellent health, while those who left school at 17 or older are more likely to report good or excellent health.

A further note of caution is that the coefficients on the explanatory variables tell us about the impact of changing each variable, *holding all of the others constant*. This means that the age variables need to be interpreted with care because the model also includes the square and the cube of age. The fact that the level of age has a negative coefficient does not mean anything in itself. In other words, it is not possible to increase age by one year without also changing the values of age-squared and age-cubed. To understand how self-assessed health changes with age, you would need to look at the change in all three variables. One way of presenting the results would be to plot the shape of the fitted polynomial function of age. An alternative approach would be to specify the age profile as a step function: in this case dummy variables could be used to indicate age ranges, 20–25, etc. Then the coefficients would indicate the impact of each age group relative to a reference age range that is omitted from the model.

The interpretation of the results so far assumes that the model we are using is well specified. For example, choosing the probit model assumes that the function F(.) is the normal distribution function and that its argument is linear in the x variables. This may not be the case. A convenient way of testing the specification of the model is to use a regression error specification test **(RESET)**. This is a general test for problems with the assumed functional form of the model, in particular the assumption of linearity. It is sometimes also used as a test for omitted variables – other explanatory variables that have not been included in the model and are correlated with both the dependent variable and with the included explanatory variables. But it will only be an effective diagnostic for omitted variables if these lead to nonlinearity in the relationship between y and x.

The RESET test is easy to implement. It involves saving the predicted values from the regression function, taking the square of those values and re-estimating the model with this new variable added as an extra explanatory variable. (Higher-order terms, such as the cubed and quartic of the fitted values, could be added as well. The square is the default when the RESET test is computed automatically in Stata.) If the model is well specified, this new test variable should not be significant. If the model is poorly specified the test variable will be significant. A convenient way of carrying out the test is to look at either the t-ratio or the F test for the null hypothesis that the coefficient on the new variable equals zero (note that the t-ratio squared equals the F test). For the linear probability model of self-assessed health, reported in Table 3.1, the RESET test gives an F test statistic of 4.42 (p = 0.04). This fails a conventional 5% significance test and the size of the statistic is a cause for a concern.

Results for the probit model

How do the results for the linear probability model compare to those for the probit and logit models? Table 3.2 shows the estimates for the probit model, computed using the method of maximum likelihood estimation. Like the linear probability model, the table includes coefficients, their standard errors and z-ratios. The z-ratio is computed in the same way as the t-ratio, by taking the ratio of the coefficient and the standard error. Hypothesis testing in models estimated by maximum likelihood has to rely on the sample size being large enough for the coefficients to follow a normal distribtion (a so-called **asymptotic property**). With a large sample size the z-ratio has a standard normal distribution.

The interpretation of the probit coefficients is different from the linear probability model. Recall that the probit model takes a linear function of the explanatory variables and applies a nonlinear transformation, in this case using the 'S' curve of the normal distribution function. The coefficients relate to the underlying linear index. These are often interpreted in terms of the latent variable y*. But y* is inherently unobservable and is not measured in any kind of natural units, unlike the probability of participation. In themselves, the coefficients should therefore be interpreted only as qualitative effects. So, for example, a negative coefficient means that somebody is less likely to be a participant, and a positive coefficient means they are more likely to be a participant. Unemployment has a coefficient of −0.137 in the probit model. This cannot be compared directly to the coefficient from the linear probability model. The qualitative interpretation is that, due to the negative coefficient, the unemployed are less likely to report good or excellent health. Similarly, the qualitative results show that those in professional and managerial occupations are more likely to report good or excellent health, while those in semi-skilled and unskilled occupations are less likely to report good or excellent health. Also, those with more education are more likely to report good health and those with fewer years of education are less likely (with the possible exception of those who left school at age 19 or more).

Table 3.2: Probit model of sah

Probit estimates

Number of obs = 8895
LR chi2(27) = 401.12
Prob > chi2 = 0.0000

Log likelihood = −5116.0659

Pseudo R2 = 0.0377

yvar	Coef.	Std.Err.	z	P>|z|	[95% Conf. Interval]	
male	.0259246	.0349187	0.74	0.458	−.0425147	.094364
age	−.0090254	.0023664	−3.81	0.000	−.0136634	−.0043873
age2	−.0367239	.0085666	−4.29	0.000	−.0535141	−.0199338
age3	.1365391	.028456	4.80	0.000	.0807664	.1923118
ethbawi	−.3066757	.1349111	−2.27	0.023	−.5710966	.−0422549
ethipb	−.2609027	.1178873	−2.21	0.027	−.4919575	−.0298479
ethothnw	−.3625705	.1654855	−2.19	0.028	−.6869162	−.0382248
part	.1652719	.0535621	3.09	0.002	.0602922	.2702517
unemp	−.1370677	.0661254	−2.07	0.038	−.266671	−.0074643
retd	.0361686	.0635569	0.57	0.569	−.0884006	.1607378
stdnt	.1221332	.1516553	0.81	0.421	−.1751057	.4193722
keephse	−.0800694	.0506691	−1.58	0.114	−.179379	.0192402
lsch14u	−.2164274	.085988	−2.52	0.012	−.3849608	−.047894
lsch14	−.2203339	.0532942	−4.13	0.000	−.3247886	−.1158793
lsch15	−.1453882	.0437683	−3.32	0.001	−.2311724	−.0596039
lsch17	.0544842	.0597137	0.91	0.362	−.0625526	.1715209
lsch18	.2686861	.0650129	4.13	0.000	.1412631	.3961091
lsch19	−.0170855	.1317568	−0.13	0.897	−.2753242	.2411531
regscls	.286181	.0766413	3.73	0.000	.1359668	.4363951
regsc2	.2349733	.0424138	5.54	0.000	.1518438	.3181028
regsc3n	.1022324	.0465856	2.19	0.028	.0109263	.1935386
regsc4	−.0698505	.041477	−1.68	0.092	−.1511439	.0114429
regsc5n	−.1915523	.0604116	−3.17	0.002	−.3099569	−.0731477
widow	−.1507873	.0571748	−2.64	0.008	−.2628478	−.0387269
single	−.0850688	.049903	−1.70	0.088	−.1828769	.0127393
seprd	−.2498267	.0966871	−2.58	0.010	−.43933	−.0603233
divorce	−.2015977	.0743637	−2.71	0.007	−.3473478	−.0558476
_cons	.7248271	.0536818	13.50	0.000	.6196127	.8300416

To interpret the quantitative implications of the results we need to compute **partial effects**, using **marginal effects** for continuous explanatory variables and **average effects** for binary explanatory variables. Unlike the linear probability model, the marginal or average effects are not given by the coefficients directly, but they can be computed from them. The formula for the marginal effect of an explanatory variable x_k is:

$$\partial P(y = 1|x)/\partial x_k = \beta_k f(x\beta), \tag{3}$$

where $f(.) = \partial F(.)/\partial(x\beta)$. The formula for the average effect of a binary variable is:

$$P(y = 1|x_k = 1) - P(y = 1|x_k = 0) = F(x\beta|x_k = 1) - F(x\beta|x_k = 0). \tag{4}$$

These are more complex formulae than the linear probability model due to the nonlinearity of the $F(.)$ curve. Also, it should be clear that both the marginal and average effects depend on the values of the x variables. In other words, they are different for different types of individual. The size of the effect of a variable, say unemployment, will depend on the value of the other explanatory variables, such as education, marital status and age. One common way of dealing with this is to evaluate the effect at the sample mean of the other x variables, treating this as a 'typical' observation. This is the approach adopted in software packages such as Limdep and Stata. However, this can be a rather artificial approach, especially when the x-values include dummy variables, as the typical observation is unlikely to correspond to any actual observation. An alternative is to compute the effect for each observation, using their specific x-values, and then report summary statistics such at the sample mean of the effects; this is known as the average partial effect (APE).

Table 3.3 presents the average and marginal effects for the probit model as computed automatically by the *dprobit* command in Stata. The effects in Table 3.3 can be given a quantitative interpretation and are measured in units of probability. Consider the impact of unemployment. Here the average effect is –0.047, which is very similar to the estimate of –0.045 of the linear probability model (*see* Table 3.1). It tells us that the probability of an unemployed person reporting good or excellent health is 0.047 less than a full-time employed person (at the average value of the other regressors). In this case, the estimated effect of unemployment is quite similar across the linear probability and probit specifications. However, comparing the estimates for other explanatory variables shows that this is not always the case. For example, the average effect of being in part-time, rather than full-time, work is 0.053 in the probit model (Table 3.3) compared with 0.064 in the linear probability model (Table 3.1). One note of caution is that the automated computation of partial effects provided by the *dprobit* command may produce misleading results. Table 3.3 displays separate marginal effects for age, age-squared and age-cubed, treating them as separate variables. But, of course, it is not possible to change one of these variables without changing the other two. The correct approach would be to compute the overall derivative with respect to age. A similar issue arises when interaction terms between different regressors are included in the model, and again derivatives should be computed directly.

Table 3.3: Partial effects for probit model of sah

Probit estimates

Number of obs = 8895
LR chi2(27) = 401.12
Prob > chi2 = 0.0000

Log likelihood = −5116.0659

Pseudo R2 = 0.0377

yvar	dF/dx	Std. Err.	z	P >|z|	x-bar	[95% C.I.]	
male*	.0086665	.0116609	0.74	0.458	.434401	−.014188	.031521
age	−.0030203	.0007916	−3.81	0.000	.83946	−.004572	−.001469
age2	−.0122893	.002865	−4.29	0.000	3.13702	−.017905	−.006674
age3	.0456916	.0095162	4.80	0.000	.242169	.02704	.064343
ethbawi*	−.1105744	.0515425	−2.27	0.023	.010455	−.211596	−.009553
ethipb*	−.0931605	.0443748	−2.21	0.027	.01439	−.180133	−.006187
ethothnw*	−.1321513	.0641797	−2.19	0.028	.007307	−.257941	−.006361
part*	.0531546	.0164963	3.09	0.002	.121529	.020822	.085487
unemp*	−.0474578	.0236162	−2.07	0.038	.05059	−.093745	−.001171
retd*	.0120303	.0210101	0.57	0.569	.221248	−.029149	.053209
stdnt*	.0393671	.0469502	0.81	0.421	.011804	−.052654	.131388
keephse*	−.0272401	.0175111	−1.58	0.114	.139966	−.061561	.007081
lsch14u*	−.0763619	.0317401	−2.52	0.012	.036875	−.138571	−.014153
lsch14*	−.0759303	.018846	−4.13	0.000	.252839	−.112868	−.038993
lsch15*	−.0495614	.0151727	−3.32	0.001	.271951	−.079299	−.019823
lsch17*	.017986	.0194367	0.91	0.362	.088477	−.020109	.056081
lsch18*	.0835677	.0185724	4.13	0.000	.088477	.047167	.119969
lsch19*	−.0057455	.0445217	−0.13	0.897	.013491	−.093006	.081515
regsc1s*	.0879753	.0213358	3.73	0.000	.056886	.046158	.129793
regsc2*	.0754063	.0129869	5.54	0.000	.223834	.049952	.10086
regsc3n*	.0334431	.0148789	2.19	0.028	.140866	.004281	.062605
regsc4*	−.0236895	.0142495	−1.68	0.092	.167285	−.051618	.004239
regsc5n*	−.0670684	.0220073	−3.17	0.002	.060371	−.110202	−.023935
widow*	−.0522256	.0204307	−2.64	0.008	.085779	−.092269	−.012182
single*	−.0289269	.0172294	−1.70	0.088	.17077	−.062696	.004842
seprd*	−.0889232	.0362115	−2.58	0.010	.021585	−.159897	−.01795
divorce*	−.0708975	.0272959	−2.71	0.007	.037549	−.124396	−.017399

obs. P	.714896						
pred. P	.7233723 (at x-bar)						

(*) dF/dx is for discrete change of dummy variable from 0 to 1
z and P >\|z\| are the test of the underlying coefficient being 0

. * RESET test;
chi2(1) = 0.27
Prob > chi2 = 0.6031

Finally, Table 3.3 presents the RESET test for the probit model. Unlike the linear probability model, there is no evidence of mis-specification and the chi-squared statistic for the test is 0.27 with a p-value well above conventional significance levels (p = 0.603).

Results for the logit model

Tables 3.4 and 3.5 present the coefficient estimates and average and marginal effects for a logit model of self-assessed health. Here, the standard normal distribution of the probit model is replaced by a standard logistic function. Once again, the coefficients can be given a qualitative interpretation and these qualitative effects follow the same pattern as the probit model. In the logit model, the β coefficients can be interpreted in terms of log-odds ratios, a concept that is commonly used in biostatistics and epidemiology. Because of the particular functional form of the standard logistic distribution, the odds ratio simplifies to $P(y_j = 1)/P(y_i = 0) = \exp(x\beta_j)$ and therefore the coefficients can be interpreted in terms of changes in the log-odds ratio $\log(P(y_j = 1)/P(y_i = 0))$.

The marginal and average effects show the quantitative impact, and these can be compared directly to the linear probability and probit estimates. So, for example, the average effect of unemployment in the logit model is -0.046 (Table 3.5) compared with -0.047 for the probit model (Table 3.3) and -0.045 for the linear probability model (Table 3.1). The logit model also passes a RESET test with a chi-squared statistic of 0.08 (p = 0.783).

Table 3.4: Logit model of sah

Logit estimates				Number of obs = 8895		
				LR chi2(27) = 401.74		
				Prob > chi2 = 0.0000		
Log likelihood = −5115.757				Pseudo R2 = 0.0378		

yvar	Coef.	Std. Err.	z	P >|z|	[95% Conf. Interval]	
male	.0458014	.0582573	0.79	0.432	−.0683807	.1599835
age	−.0152439	.0039875	−3.82	0.000	−.0230592	−.0074286
age2	−.061195	.0143183	−4.27	0.000	−.0892584	−.0331316
age3	.2266146	.0477364	4.75	0.000	.133053	.3201761
ethbawi	−.5069956	.2188338	−2.32	0.021	−.935902	−.0780891
ethipb	−.4397762	.1944995	−2.26	0.024	−.8209882	−.0585642
ethothnw	−.6155907	.2739546	−2.25	0.025	−1.152532	−.0786495
part	.2914546	.0915696	3.18	0.001	.1119815	.4709278
unemp	−.2224889	.1086193	−2.05	0.041	−.4353788	−.0095989
retd	.0717155	.1051686	0.68	0.495	−.134411	.2778421
stdnt	.2235216	.2682633	0.83	0.405	−.3022649	.7493081
keephse	−.1366631	.0844388	−1.62	0.106	−.3021601	.028834
lsch14u	−.3551048	.141217	−2.51	0.012	−.631885	−.0783246
lsch14	−.3648383	.0896087	−4.07	0.000	−.5404682	−.1892084
lsch15	−.2420453	.0740448	−3.27	0.001	−.3871705	−.0969201
lsch17	.0929873	.1026102	0.91	0.365	−.1081249	.2940996
lsch18	.4843371	.1163431	4.16	0.000	.2563088	.7123653
lsch19	−.01383	.2273481	−0.06	0.951	−.4594241	.431764
regsc1s	.5064417	.1361412	3.72	0.000	.2396098	.7732735
regsc2	.4019567	.0724685	5.55	0.000	.259921	.5439925
regsc3n	.1699224	.0780869	2.18	0.030	.0168749	.3229699
regsc4	−.1159152	.0679944	−1.70	0.088	−.2491818	.0173515
regsc5n	−.3075666	.098354	−3.13	0.002	−.5003369	−.1147963
widow	−.2458365	.0932408	−2.64	0.008	−.4285852	−.0630878
single	−.1457644	.0835879	−1.74	0.081	−.3095937	.0180649
seprd	−.4221802	.1570441	−2.69	0.007	−.729981	−.1143794
divorce	−.3323718	.1225983	−2.71	0.007	−.57266	−.0920835
_cons	1.178291	.0903083	13.05	0.000	1.00129	1.355292

Table 3.5: Partial effects for logit model of sah

variable	dy/dx	X
male*	.0091059	.434401
age	−.0030348	.839460
age2	−.012183	3.13702
age3	.0451156	.242169
ethbawi*	−.1110924	.010455
ethipb*	−.0952794	.014390
ethothnw*	−.1371255	.007307
part*	.0550491	.121529
unemp*	−.0462216	.050590
retd*	.0141476	.221248
stdnt*	.042251	.011804
keephse*	−.0278002	.139966
lsch14u*	−.0756127	.036875
lsch15*	−.0493459	.271951
lsch17*	.018189	.088477
lsch18*	.087384	.088477
lsch19*	−.0027617	.013491
regscls*	.0901681	.056886
regsc2*	.0758616	.223834
regsc3n*	.0328796	.140866
regsc4*	−.0234723	.167285
regsc5n*	−.0647758	.060371
widow	−.0489424	.085779
single	−.0290195	.170770
seprd	−.0840498	.021585
divorce	−.0661703	.037549

(*) dy/dx is for discrete change of dummy variable from 0 to 1

. * RESET test;
chi2(1) = 0.08
Prob > chi2 = 0.7826

Appendix: Stata code for binary choice models

Linear probability model

The basic linear probability model can be estimated by ordinary least squares (OLS) using the 'regress' command. Robust standard errors are used. Also the 'predict' command is used to save the fitted values from the linear regression as a new variable called 'yf':

```
regress yvar $xvars, robust
predict yf
```

For comparison with the probit and logit models it is useful to save and rename the coefficients. Here the coefficient on 'unemp' is singled-out and saved as a scalar 'bun_lpm':

```
matrix blpm=e(b)
matrix list blpm
scalar bun_lpm=_b[unemp]
scalar list bun_lpm
```

The fitted values, saved above as the new variable 'yf', can be used to create the weights that are needed to adjust for the heteroskedasticity that is inherent in the linear probability model. Then the 'aweight' option can be used to run weighted least squares (WLS):

```
* WEIGHTED LEAST SQUARES
gen wt=1/(yf*(1-yf))
regress yvar $xvars [aweight=wt]
```

The fitted values can be squared and added back to the original regression model in order to compute the RESET test for mis-specification of the model. Here we are only interested in the t-ratio for the new variable 'yf2' so the rest of the regression output is suppressed using the 'quietly' option:

```
* RESET TEST
gen yf2=yf^2
quietly regress yvar $xvars yf2, robust
test yf2=0
```

Probit model

The syntax for the probit model is very similar to the linear regression, with 'regress' replaced by 'probit'. Fitted values can be saved for the linear index, $x\beta$, using 'predict':

```
probit yvar $xvars
predict yf, xb
```

Stata provides a command, 'dprobit', that automatically presents the results as partial effects, calculated at the sample means of the regressors:

```
dprobit yvar $xvars
```

Again we can save the beta coefficients and, in this case, also rescale them so that they are comparable to the linear probability model. There are two options discussed in the literature, rescaling by 1.6 or by 1.8. The code does both:

```
matrix bpbt=e(b)
matrix list bpbt
scalar bun_pbt=_b[unemp]
scalar bun_pbt18=_b[unemp]*1.8
scalar bun_pbt16=_b[unemp]*1.6
scalar list bun_pbt bun_pbt18 bun_pbt16
```

Rather than calculating partial effects at the sample means of the regressors (as in 'dprobit'), it is preferable to compute them using the actual x-values for each observation. The formulas for the marginal effect of a continuous variable and the average effect of a discrete variable can be computed directly:

```
* MARGINAL EFFECTS
gen mepbt_unemp=bun_pbt*normden(yf)
* AVERAGE EFFECTS
gen aepbt_unemp=0
replace aepbt_unemp=norm(yf+bun_pbt)-norm(yf) if unemp==0
replace aepbt_unemp=norm(yf)-norm(yf-bun_pbt) if unemp==1
```

Once these have been computed, 'summ' can be used to compute the average partial effects and other descriptive statistics. A histogram of the partial effects could be plotted using 'hist' to give a sense of the overall distribution of the effects:

```
summ mepbt_unemp aepbt_unemp
hist aepbt_unemp
```

The format for the RESET test mirrors the code used for the LPM:

```
gen yf2=yf^2
quietly probit yvar $xvars yf2
test yf2=0
```

Logit model

Most of the code needed for the logit model is analogous to the probit. There is no equivalent to 'dprobit', so the slower command 'mfx' has to be used. The expessions for the direct computation of the partial effects use the logistic distribution rather than the standard normal distribution:

```
logit yvar $xvars
mfx compute if e(sample)
predict yf, xb
* SAVE COEFFICIENTS
matrix blgt=e(b)
matrix list blgt
scalar bun_lgt=_b[unemp]
scalar list bun_lgt bun_pbt18 bun_pbt16
* MARGINAL EFFECTS
gen melgt_unemp=bun_lgt*( exp(yf)/(1+exp(yf)))*(1-exp(yf)/
(1+exp(yf)))
* AVERAGE EFFECTS
gen aelgt_unemp=0
replace aelgt_unemp=exp(yf+bun_lgt)/(1+exp(yf+bun_lgt))-
exp(yf)/(1+exp(yf)) if unemp==0
replace aelgt_unemp=exp(yf)/(1+exp(yf))-exp(yf-bun_lgt)/(1+exp(yf-
bun_lgt)) if unemp==1
summ mepbt_unemp aepbt_unemp melgt_unemp aelgt_unemp
scalar list bun_lpm
* RESET TEST
gen yf2=yf^2
quietly logit yvar $xvars yf2
test yf2=0
```

Chapter 4

The ordered probit model

Methods

The empirical example in the previous section uses a binary measure of self-assessed health. This variable was created artificially by collapsing the underlying four-category scale where health could be assessed as either excellent, good, fair or poor. This is an example of a categorical variable where respondents are asked to report a particular category and where there is a natural ordering. It seems reasonable to assume that excellent health is better than good, which is better than fair, which is better than poor, for everyone in the population. An econometric model that can be used to deal with ordered categorical variables is the **ordered probit** model. This is designed to model a discrete dependent variable that takes ordered multinomial outcomes. For example, $y = 0, 1, 2, 3...$ It should be stressed that y is measured on an ordinal scale and the numerical values of y are arbitrary, except that they must be in ascending order.

The ordered probit model is an extension of the binary probit model (a similar extension is available for the logit model). Like the binary probit model, the ordered probit model can be expressed in terms of an underlying latent variable y^*. Here this could be interpreted as the individual's 'true health'. The higher the value of y^*, the more likely they are to report a higher category of self-assessed health. In our case there are four categories, so the range of values y^* should be divided into four intervals, each one corresponding to a different category of self-assessed health. The threshold values (μ) correspond to the cut-offs where an individual moves from reporting one category of self-assessed health to another. It is not possible to identify both the constant term and all the cut-off points. So, in order to estimate the model, some of the threshold values have to be fixed. The lowest value is set at minus infinity, the highest value is set at plus infinity and one other value has to be fixed. Conventionally, either the upper bound of the first interval (μ_1) is set equal to zero or the constant term is excluded from the regression model. Like the binary probit model, explanatory variables are introduced into the model by making the latent variable y^* a linear function of the xs, and adding a normally distributed error term. This means that the probability of an individual reporting a particular value of $y = j$ is given by the difference between the probability of the respondent having a value of y^* less than μ_j and the probability of having a value of y^* less than μ_{j-1}. Using these probabilities it is possible to use **maximum likelihood estimation** to estimate the parameters of the model. These include the βs (the coefficients on the x variables) and the unknown cut-off values (the μs).

The ordered probit model applies when the threshold values (μ) are unknown. A variant on the model is **interval regression** (sometimes known as **grouped data regression**). This can be used when the values of thresholds are observed. For example, in many health interview surveys, including HALS, individuals are presented with a range of categories and asked to state where their income lies. These categories are selected by the researcher and the upper and lower thresholds are known. Because the values of the μs are known and do not have to be estimated, the estimates of the coefficients on the explanatory variables are more efficient. Also, because the values of the thresholds are in natural units, such as money, the predicted values from the grouped data regression are also measured in those units. This means that the grouped data regression is able to estimate the variance of the error term (σ^2) as well as the βs. What is more, this scaling means that the latent variable is also measured in natural units and hence the coefficients measure marginal or average effects in natural units.

An application to self-assessed health

To illustrate the use of the **ordered probit model**, Table 4.1 shows estimates for the four-category measure of self-assessed health. The dependent variable is coded 0 for poor health, 1 for fair health, 2 for good health and 3 for excellent health. Table 4.1 includes the coefficients, their standard errors and z-ratios. It also includes estimates of the threshold parameters μ_1, μ_2 and μ_3 (the default in Stata is to exclude the constant term in order to identify model). These are shown as _cut1, _cut2 and _cut3 and imply that a value of the latent variable less than −1.717 corresponds to poor health, a value between −1.717 and −0.641 corresponds to fair health, a value between −0.641 and 0.783 corresponds to good health, and a value above 0.783 corresponds to excellent health. Notice that the predicted value of y* for the reference individual, where all of the explanatory variables equal zero, is zero. This value lies between −0.641 and 0.783, hence the reference individual would be predicted to report good health.

As for the binary probit model, the coefficients on the explanatory variables have a qualitative interpretation. A positive coefficient means that an individual has a higher value of latent health and is more likely to report a higher category of self-assessed health. A negative value means that they have a lower value of the latent variable and are likely to report a lower category of self-assessed health. As before, the results show a socioeconomic gradient in self-assessed health. Those in professional and managerial occupational groups have positive coefficients, those in semi-skilled and unskilled occupations have negative coefficients. A similar gradient is apparent for levels of education. Because the threshold values are unknown, the latent variable and hence the coefficients are not measured in natural units. Like the binary probit model, quantitative predictions should be made on the basis of marginal effects for continuous explanatory variables and average effects for binary explanatory variables.

Once again, it is important to test the specification of the model before putting too much weight on the results. In fact (*see* Table 4.1) a RESET test suggests that the model is mis-specified, the chi-squared is 5.20 (p = 0.023). This suggests that more work needs to be done to improve the specification of the model, perhaps by changing the way in which the explanatory variables are measured, by finding additional explanatory variables, or by splitting the sample into separate groups, perhaps by gender, or using a distribution other than the standard normal.

Table 4.1: Ordered probit model of sah

Ordered probit estimates	Number of obs = 8895
	LR chi2(27) = 399.67
	Prob > chi2 = 0.0000
Log likelihood = −10163.906	Pseudo R2 = 0.0193

yvar	Coef.	Std. Err.	z	P >|z|	[95% Conf. Interval]	
male	.0628071	.0281575	2.23	0.026	.0076195	.1179948
age	−.0060561	.0018943	−3.20	0.001	−.0097689	−.0023433
age2	−.028396	.0069248	−4.10	0.000	−.0419684	−.0148237
age3	.1069476	.0228589	4.68	0.000	.0621451	.1517502
ethbawi	−.1399885	.1138824	−1.23	0.219	−.3631939	.083217
ethipb	−.1968899	.0975955	−2.02	0.044	−.3881735	−.0056063
ethothnw	−.343557	.1358343	−2.53	0.011	−.6097873	−.0773267
part	.1887253	.0419252	4.50	0.000	.1065534	.2708972
unemp	−.1069106	.0551405	−1.94	0.053	−.2149841	.0011628
retd	.0416581	.0523803	0.80	0.426	−.0610054	.1443216
stdnt	.0248111	.1165797	0.21	0.831	−.2036809	.2533031
keephse	−.0802928	.0407453	−1.97	0.049	−.1601522	−.0004334
lsch14u	−.1815896	.0715292	−2.54	0.011	−.3217843	−.0413949
lsch14	−.1952184	.0430878	−4.53	0.000	−.279669	−.1107679
lsch15	−.0857022	.034904	−2.46	0.014	−.1541127	−.0172918
lsch17	.1004313	.0464239	2.16	0.031	.0094421	.1914204
lsch18	.145202	.0474957	3.06	0.002	.0521121	.2382918
lsch19	.0597935	.1039537	0.58	0.565	−.143952	.263539
regsc1s	.2095555	.057166	3.67	0.000	.0975122	.3215989
regsc2	.2018999	.0334748	6.03	0.000	.1362904	.2675094
regsc3n	.1167197	.0376377	3.10	0.002	.0429512	.1904881
regsc4	−.0599731	.0344098	−1.74	0.081	−.1274151	.0074688
regsc5n	−.1469187	.0510459	−2.88	0.004	−.2469668	−.0468706
widow	−.1094727	.0478125	−2.29	0.022	−.2031834	−.015762
single	−.0322312	.040252	−0.80	0.423	−.1111237	.0466613
seprd	−.1818617	.0798724	−2.28	0.023	−.3384087	−.0253147
divorce	−.1846496	.0614381	−3.01	0.003	−.305066	−.0642332
_cut1	−1.717435	.0471383	(Ancillary parameters)			
_cut2	−.6412847	.0436984				
_cut3	.7830036	.0438347				

RESET
(1) yf2 = 0.0
chi2(1) = 5.20
Prob > chi2 = 0.0226

Appendix: Stata code for the ordered probit model

The basic syntax for running an ordered probit model, with an option to tablulate the actual and fitted values is given below. Predictions of the linear index are saved for future use:

```
oprobit yvar $xvars, table
predict yf, xb
```

With the ordered probit model, partial effects can be computed for each of the observed values of y. Here the partial effects for $P(y = 0)$ are computed. An automated version is available with the 'mfx' command (based on evaluating at the means of the regressors):

```
mfx compute, predict(outcome(0))
```

Or the partial effects can be computed for each observation. The formula for the average effect of 'unemp' involves the estimated cut-points, saved as scalars b[_cut1], etc., as well as the beta coefficients:

```
scalar mu1=_b[_cut1]
scalar bunemp=_b[unemp]
gen aeop_unemp=0
replace aeop_unemp=norm(mu1-yf-bunemp)-norm(mu1-yf) if unemp==0
replace aeop_unemp=norm(mu1-yf)-norm(mu1-yf+bunemp) if unemp==1
summ aeop_unemp
hist aeop_unemp
```

The RESET test follows the by now familiar format:

```
gen yf2=yf^2
quietly oprobit yvar $xvars yf2
test yf2=0
drop yf yf2
```

Chapter 5

Multinomial models

The multinomial logit model

The ordered probit model discussed in the previous section applies to ordered categorical variables. Multinomial models apply to discrete dependent variables that can take unordered multinomial outcomes, for example, y = 0, 1, 2, 3..., that represent a set of mutually exclusive choices. Again, the numerical values of y are arbitrary and in this case they do not imply any natural ordering of the outcomes. A classic example in economics is 'modal choice' in transport. Here, the outcomes could represent different modes of transport, for example plane, train, car, and the individual faces a choice of one of these mutually exclusive modes of transport. This choice will depend on characteristics of the alternatives, such as price, convenience, quality of service and so on, and the characteristics of individuals, such as their level of income. Some of the characteristics of the alternatives, such as distance to the nearest hospital, may vary across individuals as well. There is unlikely to be a natural ordering of the choices that applies to all individuals in all situations. In health economics, multinomial models are often applied to the choice of health insurance plan or of healthcare provider. They could also be used to model a choice of a particular treatment regimen for an individual patient.

The most commonly applied model is the **mixed logit** model, which is a natural extension of the binary logit model. In the mixed logit model, the probability of individual i choosing outcome j, is given by,

$$P_{ij} = \exp(x_i\beta_j + z_{ij}\gamma) \,/\, \Sigma_k \exp(x_i\beta_k + z_{ik}\gamma) \tag{5}$$

Notice that the coefficients (β_j) on the explanatory variables that vary across individuals (x_i) are allowed to vary across the choices, j. So, for example, the impact of income could be different for different types of healthcare provider. The coefficients (γ) on the variables that vary across the choices and perhaps also across individuals (z_{ij}) are constant. So, for example, there may be a common price effect on the choice of provider. The mixed logit nests two special cases: the **multinomial logit** or 'characteristics of the chooser' model, when all of the γ equal zero; and the **conditional logit** or 'characteristics of the choices' model, when all of the β_j equal zero. It is worth noting that the label 'mixed logit' is sometimes applied to the more complex random parameters logit model which is not discussed here.

Focusing on the multinomial logit model, it is not possible to identify separate βs for all of the choices. To deal with this it is conventional to set the βs for one of the outcomes equal to zero. This normalisation reflects the fact that only relative probabilities can be identified with respect to some baseline alternative. For example, in a model of hospital utilisation, where the possible outcomes are:

- no use of hospital services
- use of hospital outpatient services only
- use of hospital inpatient services and/or outpatient services

no use may be treated as the baseline category. The multinomial logit model would identify the probability of using outpatient services relative to no use and the probability of using inpatient services relative to no use.

The mixed logit model is well established and widely available in computer software packages. However, it is a restrictive specification and, in particular, it implies the 'independence of irrelevant alternatives' (IIA) property. To see this, consider the ratio of the probabilities of choosing two specific alternatives, j and l:

$$P_{ij}/P_{il} = [\exp(x_i\beta_j + z_{ij}\gamma) \ / \ \Sigma_k \exp(x_i\beta_k + z_{ik}\gamma)]/[\exp(x_i\beta_l + z_{il}\gamma) \ / \ \Sigma_k \exp(x_i\beta_k + z_{ik}\gamma)]$$

$$= \exp(x_i\beta_j + z_{ij}\gamma)/\exp(x_i\beta_l + z_{il}\gamma) \qquad (6)$$

This shows that the relative probability only depends on the coefficients and characteristics of the two choices – j and l – and not on any of the other choices available. This implies that if a new alternative is introduced, all of the absolute probabilities will be reduced proportionately. For example, consider the case of an individual choosing between a branded medicine (brand X) and a generic alternative (generic A). Let us say that, faced with this choice, the probability of choosing brand X is 0.5 and the probability of choosing generic A is 0.5. The relative probability is therefore 0.5/0.5 = 1. Now we introduce a third alternative, a new generic B, which shares the same characteristics as generic A. If the two generic drugs are perfect substitutes for each other, we might expect that the probability of choosing brand X will remain 0.5 and the probability of choosing each of the generic will be reduced to 0.25 each. But this contradicts the IIA property, as the relative probability of choosing brand X compared to generic A will be increased to 0.5/0.25 = 2. In order to satisfy the property, all of the absolute probabilities need to change so that all equal 0.333 and the relative probabilities remain constant. Many authors argue that the IIA property is too restrictive for many applications of multinomial models. The IIA property can be relaxed by using various more general alternatives: such as the nested multinomial logit, the mixed or random parameters logit or the multinomial probit specification (*see* Jones 2000 and Train 2003 for further details).

It is possible to use the mixed logit model to test whether the IIA property is appropriate. This test will work with three or more alternatives. The basic idea is to estimate the model with all of the alternatives and then to re-estimate it, dropping one or more of the alternatives. The estimated coefficients should not change when an alternative is dropped and so a comparison of the two sets of results can be used to test for the property. This is based on a **Hausman test** for whether there is a significant difference between two sets of coefficients: one set that is efficient under the null (IIA holds) but inconsistent under the alternative (IIA does not hold) and another set that is inefficient under the null but still consistent under the alternative. In this case the first set of coefficients would be taken from the model with all the alternatives included, the second from the model with an alternative excluded.

An application

The mixed logit model only applies when there is a set of mutually exclusive and exhaustive outcomes. For this application we use the data on healthcare utilisation that were added to the questionnaire at the second wave of the survey (HALS2). The HALS data on healthcare utilisation have to be recoded to satisfy the conditions of mutually exclusive and exhaustive outcomes. Here a new variable is created that has three outcomes: no use of healthcare (y = 0); a GP visit but no use of hospital visits, whether inpatient or outpatient (y = 1); a hospital visit, with or without a GP visit (y = 2). Results for the multinomial logit model applied to this dependent variable are shown in Table 5.1. These include the socioeconomic variables, measured at HALS2, as regressors. Note that the model includes the usual list of regressors, which does not have explicit measures of morbidity. The impact of morbidity on the use of healthcare is likely to be picked up by age and gender (which are strongly statistically significant in the model) and to some extent by socioeconomic characteristics that are linked to health.

Table 5.1: Multinomial logit model of healthcare use at HALS2

Multinomial logistic regression

Number of obs = 5345
LR chi2(54) = 195.10
Prob > chi2 = 0.0000

Log likelihood = −4509.0832

Pseudo R2 = 0.0212

use	Coef.	Std. Err.	z	P >|z|	[95% Conf. Interval]	
1						
male	−.3710599	.0810458	−4.58	0.000	−.5299067	−.212213
age	−.1648649	.0771253	−2.14	0.033	−.3160276	−.0137021
age2	.354964	.1441615	2.46	0.014	.0724127	.6375153
age3	−.2167922	.0840693	−2.58	0.010	−.381565	−.0520194
ethbawi	−.5399794	.4968079	−1.09	0.277	−1.513705	.4337462
ethipb	.3084649	.3323884	0.93	0.353	−.3430044	.9599342
ethothnw	−1.19211	.7415567	−1.61	0.108	−2.645535	.261314
part	.0108215	.111776	0.10	0.923	−.2082555	.2298985
unemp	.0522356	.2288557	0.23	0.819	−.3963133	.5007846
retd	−.0497801	.1493546	−0.33	0.739	−.3425097	.2429496
stdnt	.6572269	.4360607	1.51	0.132	−.1974365	1.51189
keephse	.1207467	.1404428	0.86	0.390	−.1545161	.3960095
lsch14u	.2781795	.2170767	1.28	0.200	−.1472831	.703642
lsch14	.2334741	.1266671	1.84	0.065	−.014789	.4817371
lsch15	.2672454	.104424	2.56	0.010	.0625781	.4719127
lsch17	.1183566	.1413804	0.84	0.403	−.1587439	.3954571
lsch18	.0195781	.1491224	0.13	0.896	−.2726964	.3118525
lsch19	−.0324339	.3472616	−0.09	0.926	−.7130541	.6481863
regsc1s	−.1836389	.1648901	−1.11	0.265	−.5068175	.1395397
regsc2	−.1024984	.0980101	−1.05	0.296	−.2945946	.0895978
regsc3n	.0389298	.1166864	0.33	0.739	−.1897714	.267631
regsc4	.0867052	.1043228	0.83	0.406	−.1177637	.2911742
regsc5n	.2312321	.1471503	1.57	0.116	−.0571771	.5196413
widow	−.0162418	.1239365	−0.13	0.896	−.2591528	.2266692
single	−.0644249	.1374494	−0.47	0.639	−.3338209	.204971
seprd	.3342608	.2408134	1.39	0.165	−.1377249	.8062464
divorce	.0991702	.1513485	0.66	0.512	−.1974674	.3958077
_cons	.8597914	1.292219	0.67	0.506	−1.672911	3.392494

Table 5.1: (Continued)

use	Coef.	Std. Err.	z	P >|z|	[95% Conf. Interval]	
2						
male	−.3212293	.0991184	−3.24	0.001	−.5154977	−.1269608
age	−.1575255	.0943892	−1.67	0.095	−.342525	.0274739
age2	.3253331	.1769703	1.84	0.066	−.0215224	.6721885
age3	−.1939281	.1033172	−1.88	0.061	−.396426	.0085698
ethbawi	.3527783	.4347653	0.81	0.417	−.499346	1.204903
ethipb	−.2229233	.4856916	−0.46	0.646	−1.174861	.7290148
ethothnw	.0170081	.5489996	0.03	0.975	−1.059011	1.093028
part	−.3603159	.1500899	−2.40	0.016	−.6544867	−.0661452
unemp	.4250635	.242184	1.76	0.079	−.0496084	.8997355
retd	−.1779357	.1862228	−0.96	0.339	−.5429256	.1870542
stdnt	.0045098	.6343637	0.01	0.994	−1.23882	1.24784
keephse	.1555238	.1693613	0.92	0.358	−.1764182	.4874659
lsch14u	.1959821	.2806971	0.70	0.485	−.354174	.7461383
lsch14	.3985299	.155586	2.56	0.010	.0935868	.7034729
lsch15	.1824894	.1301538	1.40	0.161	−.0726073	.4375862
lsch17	.0072374	.1775626	0.04	0.967	−.3407789	.3552538
lsch18	.0025037	.1834829	0.01	0.989	−.3571163	.3621236
lsch19	.3461163	.3645636	0.95	0.342	−.3684152	1.060648
regscls	−.2300271	.2129076	−1.08	0.280	−.6473184	.1872641
regsc2	.033787	.1190705	0.28	0.777	−.1995868	.2671608
regsc3n	.1012446	.1423716	0.71	0.477	−.1777985	.3802877
regsc4	.0780057	.1291655	0.60	0.546	−.175154	.3311654
regsc5n	−.2238345	.2066197	−1.08	0.279	−.6288016	.1811326
widow	.0153144	.1533987	0.10	0.920	−.2853415	.3159703
single	−.0542009	.1660829	−0.33	0.744	−.3797174	.2713157
seprd	.2653849	.3040131	0.87	0.383	−.3304699	.8612397
divorce	.2863276	.175175	1.63	0.102	−.057009	.6296643
_cons	.4226484	1.574012	0.27	0.788	−2.662359	3.507656

(Outcome use==0 is the comparison group)

To identify the coefficients of the multinomial logit model one of the outcomes has to be fixed as a reference point. All of the results should be interpreted relative to this reference outcome (by default in Stata this is the case of y = 0). So they tell us about the relative probability of having a GP visit (y = 1) or a hospital visit (y = 2) rather than having no visit. The β coefficients can be interpreted in terms of log-odds ratios. Given the normalising restriction that $\beta_0 = 0$ which is required to identify the model, then the odds ratio simplifies to $P(y_j = 1)/P(y_0 = 1) = \exp(x\beta_j)$ and therefore the coefficients can be interpreted in terms of changes in the log-odds ratio $\log(P(y_j = 1)/P(y_0 = 1))$. The qualitative interpretation of the coefficients depends on their signs. So, for example, male – with a negative sign in both equations – implies that men are less likely to use GPs (y = 1) than to have no visits (y = 0) and are less likely to have a hospital visit (y = 2) than to have no visits. Overall the coefficients on the variables other than age and gender tend not to be statistically significant, but it would be important to test them in groups, for example for marital status as a whole.

Appendix: Stata code for the multinomial logit model

The multinomial logit model only applies when there is a set of mutually exclusive and exhaustive outcomes. The HALS data on healthcare utilisation have to be recoded to satisfy these conditions. Here a new variable 'use' is created, which has three outcomes: no use of healthcare ($y = 0$); a GP visit but no use of hospital visits, whether inpatient or outpatient ($y = 1$); a hospital visit, with or without a GP visit ($y = 2$). The command takes account of missing values which are coded as '.' in Stata:

```
gen hosp=hospop==1 | hospip==1
gen use = 0
replace use=1 if visitgp==1 & hosp==0
replace use=2 if hosp==1
replace use=. if visitgp==.
replace yvar=use
```

Estimates of the multinomial logit model can be obtained from the 'mlogit' command:

```
mlogit yvar $xvars
```

To check whether the independence of irrelevant alternatives (IIA) property holds, it is possible to run a **Hausman test** procedure. This compares the general model estimated above with a restricted model in which one of the categories ($y = 2$ in this case) is dropped:

```
* Hausman test of IIA
est store hall
mlogit yvar $xvars if yvar!=2
est store hpartial
hausman hpartial hall, alleqs constant
```

The same routine could be run again dropping other alternatives.

Chapter 6

The bivariate probit model

Methods

The ordered and multinomial models discussed in the previous two sections deal with dependent variables that can have different categorical outcomes. However, in both cases, there is a single underlying outcome variable. In contrast, the **bivariate probit** model provides a way of dealing with two separate binary dependent variables. Essentially it takes two independent binary probit models and estimates them together, allowing for a correlation between the error term of the two equations. The practical application discussed here uses the HALS data to estimate the probability of someone reporting 'good' or 'excellent' self-assessed health together with the probability of them being a current smoker. Allowing for correlation between the error terms of the two equations recognises that there may be unobservable characteristics of individuals that influence *both* whether they smoke and their self-assessed health.

Given that the bivariate probit model is a natural extension of the binary probit model, it is possible to think about the bivariate model in terms of two latent variables, say, y^*_1 and y^*_2. Each of the latent variables is assumed to be a linear function of a set of explanatory variables, which may or may not be the same for the two equations, and each equation contains an error term. Like the binary probit model, these error terms are assumed to be normally distributed, but they come from a joint or bivariate normal distribution. The bivariate distribution allows for a non-zero correlation between the errors. In other words, it is not assumed that the two error terms are independent of each other.

With two binary variables four possible outcomes can be observed. In the example here, the possible outcomes are: a smoker who reports good or excellent health; a smoker who reports poor or fair health; a non-smoker who reports good or excellent health; or a non-smoker who reports fair or poor health. These correspond to different values of the latent variables y^*_1 and y^*_2 (remember that y^* is positive for a participant and non-positive for a non-participant). Using the assumption that the error terms are bivariate normal, it is possible to write down the probability of each of these four outcomes as a function of the explanatory variables and the unknown parameters of the model. This allows the model to be estimated by **maximum likelihood** methods. Because the outcomes are estimated jointly, it is possible to identify not only the slope coefficients for each of the two sets of explanatory variables but also the coefficient of correlation between the two error terms (ρ).

As with the **binary probit** model, the latent variables – and hence the βs – are not measured in natural units and can only be given a qualitative interpretation but, like the binary probit model, marginal and average effects can be calculated. There is now a range of options for interpreting the results. First, the same formulae as used for the binary probit marginal and average effects can be used for the bivariate probit. This gives the impact of a change of one of the explanatory variables on the marginal probability of each outcome, for example the probability of someone being a smoker, or the probability of someone being in good or excellent health. Second, it is possible to calculate the marginal effect of an explanatory variable on the joint probability of each of the four outcome combinations, for example the probability that an individual is both a smoker and in good or excellent health. Finally, it is possible to calculate the marginal effects of the explanatory variables on conditional probabilities, for example the probability that someone reports good or excellent health, given that they are a smoker.

An application to smoking and health

Table 6.1 shows the results for the bivariate probit model of smoking and self-assessed health estimated using the same set of explanatory variables as before. The coefficient estimates for both equations are broadly similar to those obtained using binary probit models. The equation for regular smoking (y2) shows that those in professional and managerial socioeconomic groups are less likely to be smokers, while those in unskilled manual occupations are more likely to be smokers. Similarly, those who left school at 18 are less likely to be smokers, while those who left school before 16 are more likely to be smokers. The socio-economic gradient is once again apparent for self-assessed health (y1), with those in professional and managerial occupations more likely to report good or excellent health and those in unskilled and semi-skilled occupations less likely to report good or excellent health. The new information provided by the bivariate probit model is the estimate of ρ, the correlation coefficient for the two error terms. The estimate is −0.172 and the chi-squared test of 84.06 shows that this estimate is significantly different from zero. This is a plausible result that indicates that unobservable factors that are positively related to smoking are negatively related to good health.

Table 6.1: Bivariate probit model of smoking and sah

Bivariate probit regression				Number of obs = 8895		
				Wald chi2(54) = 961.06		
Log likelihood = −10380.573				Prob > chi2 = 0.0000		

	Coef.	Std. Err.	z	P >|z|	[95% Conf. Interval]	
y1 (SAH)						
male	.0287978	.0348825	0.83	0.409	−.0395705	.0971662
age	−.0090962	.002365	−3.85	0.000	−.0137314	−.0044609
age2	−.0365567	.0085641	−4.27	0.000	−.0533421	−.0197714
age3	.1362723	.0284205	4.79	0.000	.0805691	.1919755
ethbawi	−.3057385	.1346342	−2.27	0.023	−.5696167	−.0418603
ethipb	−.2643758	.1175324	−2.25	0.024	−.494735	−.0340166
ethothnw	−.3633282	.1653823	−2.20	0.028	−.6874715	−.0391849
part	.1670081	.0535211	3.12	0.002	.0621088	.2719075
unemp	−.1389813	.066009	−2.11	0.035	−.2683565	−.009606
retd	.0366801	.0634862	0.58	0.563	−.0877505	.1611108
stdnt	.1194236	.1519335	0.79	0.432	−.1783606	.4172079
keephse	−.0774881	.0506601	−1.53	0.126	−.1767802	.021804
lsch14u	−.2147689	.0859358	−2.50	0.012	−.3832	−.0463379
lsch14	−.2191826	.053261	−4.12	0.000	−.3235723	−.114793

Table 6.1: (Continued)

	Coef.	Std. Err.	z	P >|z|	[95% Conf. Interval]	
lsch15	−.1452899	.0437732	−3.32	0.001	−.2310839	−.059496
lsch17	.05568	.0597649	0.93	0.352	−.061457	.172817
lsch18	.2667823	.064975	4.11	0.000	.1394336	.3941309
lsch19	−.0177439	.1317902	−0.13	0.893	−.2760479	.2405602
regsc1s	.2906421	.0768606	3.78	0.000	.1399981	.441286
regsc2	.2364005	.0424117	5.57	0.000	.1532751	.3195259
regsc3n	.1023298	.0465678	2.20	0.028	.0110585	.1936011
regsc4	−.069094	.0414707	−1.67	0.096	−.1503751	.0121871
regsc5n	−.1918154	.0603343	−3.18	0.001	−.3100684	−.0735623
widow	−.15092	.0570616	−2.64	0.008	−.2627586	−.0390814
single	−.0861691	.0498545	−1.73	0.084	−.183882	.0115439
seprd	−.2501239	.0966591	−2.59	0.010	−.4395722	−.0606755
divorce	−.2027916	.074228	−2.73	0.006	−.3482757	−.0573074
_cons	.722309	.0536319	13.47	0.000	.6171923	.8274257
y2 (SMOKE)						
male	.0553883	.0346972	1.60	0.110	−.0126169	.1233935
age	−.0081113	.0023966	−3.38	0.001	−.0128086	−.0034141
age2	−.03637	.0085135	−4.27	0.000	−.0530562	−.0196838
age3	−.0504658	.03064	−1.65	0.100	−.1105191	.0095876
ethbawi	−.3310786	.1431177	−2.31	0.021	−.6115841	−.0505731
ethipb	−.2997154	.1261894	−2.38	0.018	−.5470421	−.0523888
ethothnw	.1957156	.1649357	1.19	0.235	−.1275523	.5189835
part	−.0694085	.0509684	−1.36	0.173	−.1693047	.0304876
unemp	.3847182	.0650261	5.92	0.000	.2572693	.5121671
retd	.0583059	.065077	0.90	0.370	−.0692427	.1858545
stdnt	−.2108295	.1557235	−1.35	0.176	−.516042	.094383
keephse	.0046992	.0493621	0.10	0.924	−.0920488	.1014472
lsch14u	.2546079	.0907126	2.81	0.005	.0768143	.4324014
lsch14	.2478051	.0540179	4.59	0.000	.141932	.3536782
lsch15	.2215362	.0422187	5.25	0.000	.1387892	.3042833
lsch17	.0089813	.057649	0.16	0.876	−.1040086	.1219713
lsch18	−.2461978	.0614527	−4.01	0.000	−.366643	−.1257527
lsch19	−.0484965	.1319448	−0.37	0.713	−.3071036	.2101106
regsc1s	−.507897	.0770645	−6.59	0.000	−.6589406	−.3568533
regsc2	−.2822696	.0412017	−6.85	0.000	−.3630233	−.2015158
regsc3n	−.2360586	.0463523	−5.09	0.000	−.3269074	−.1452097
regsc4	.0407858	.0411539	0.99	0.322	−.0398744	.121446
regsc5n	.1580333	.0607571	2.60	0.009	.0389515	.277115
widow	.0672059	.0612781	1.10	0.273	−.0528969	.1873087
single	.0568438	.0492002	1.16	0.248	−.0395869	.1532744
seprd	.397851	.095015	4.19	0.000	.2116251	.584077
divorce	.3727787	.0722291	5.16	0.000	.2312123	.5143452
_cons	−.4207566	.0521887	−8.06	0.000	−.5230446	−.3184686
/athrho	−.1736459	.0190506	−9.11	0.000	−.2109844	−.1363073
rho	−.1719214	.0184875			−.2079086	−.1354694

Likelihood ratio test of rho=0:   chi2(1) = 84.0588 Prob > chi2 = 0.0000

Appendix: Stata code for the bivariate probit model

The bivariate probit model requires two binary dependent variables. Here we use indicators of regular smoking ('regfag') and of excellent or good self-assessed health ('sah'):

```
gen yvar1=regfag
gen yvar2=sah
```

The simple form of the model uses the same set of regressors in both equations. Predictions of the linear index are saved for each equation:

```
biprobit yvar1 yvar2 $xvars
predict yf1, xb1
predict yf2, xb2
```

Partial effects can be computed for the marginal, conditional and joint distributions. To illustrate, the following code computes the average effect of 'unemp' on the marginal probability of being a smoker, p(regfag = 1). The results are summarised and displayed in a histogram:

```
scalar bun_pbt=_b[yvar1:unemp]
gen aepbt_unemp=0
replace aepbt_unemp=norm(yf1+bun_pbt)-norm(yf1) if unemp==0
replace aepbt_unemp=norm(yf1)-norm(yf1-bun_pbt) if unemp==1
summ aepbt_unemp
hist aepbt_unemp
```

Chapter 7

The selection problem

Identification

Sample selection bias arises when there are missing data for the dependent variable of interest. Recall the discussion of **item non-response** in the introduction. For example, in the HALS data set, measures of physiological health were collected at the nurse visit, but not all of the original interviewees agreed to participate in the nurse visit. Models of measured health outcomes (for example forced expiratory volume, *fev*) could be estimated on the sample of individuals who responded to the nurse visit. But the selection problem means that it may not be possible to make inferences about the determinants of health outcome in the population as a whole. If there are systematic differences between the type of individuals who respond and those who do not, analysts are faced with a fundamental problem of identification.

For each individual in the HALS data set, we know whether or not they responded to the nurse visit, and we know the characteristics of those who responded and those who did not. Also we have a measure of the health outcome for those who responded and their associated characteristics. This means we could estimate the probability of responding, conditional on the explanatory variables, and we can estimate the expected value of *fev*, conditional upon the characteristics and on the fact that the individual agreed to participate. The identification problem arises because there is no way of knowing the *fev* score that would have been reported by any individual who refused to participate in the nurse visit. They could have reported any logically feasible value of *fev*. The fact that it is not possible to observe the outcome of the non-responders means that, in general, it is not possible to identify the expected value of the outcome in the population as a whole. In other words, it is not possible to identify the population regression function, $E(y|x)$.

At a fundamental level this identification problem is insurmountable. However, inferences can be made if the analyst is willing to impose some assumptions on their model and data. Traditionally, the statistical literature often assumes independence or ignorable non-response. This is a strong assumption, which asserts that those individuals who do not respond would behave in the same way as those who do respond, conditional upon the observed explanatory variables. Given this assumption, estimates can be adjusted for non-response using **inverse probability weights**, a method that is discussed in more detail in Chapters 8 and 11.

Not only is ignorability a strong assumption, it is not possible to test its validity. In the kind of observational health surveys often used in health economics it is often likely to be untenable. For example, the reasons why an individual decides not to participate in the nurse visit may be correlated with unobservable factors that also influence their health outcome. This would violate the assumption of ignorable non-response and lead to potential selection bias. Participating in the nurse visit is time-consuming and it may be that those who suspect they may benefit more from the visit, due to pre-existing chronic conditions, may be more willing to take part. Of course, this also means that their health outcomes are likely to be poorer than for those who are not willing to participate.

The selection problem can be dealt with if the analyst is willing to impose identifying restrictions on their model. This involves making assumptions about the functional form of the regression model, possibly excluding some explanatory variables that predict non-response from the equations that predict the outcome variable, and also assumptions about the distribution of the error terms in the two equations. In the econometrics literature the traditional approach to the selection problem has been a parametric approach, based on the so-called **Heckit** model, first introduced by James Heckman (*see*, for example, Heckman 1979). This uses linear regression equations and assumes that the error terms have a normal distribution. However, recent years have seen the development of less restrictive semi-parametric estimators which relax some, though not all, of the identifying restrictions (*see* Jones 2000).

The Heckit model

The sample selection model consists of two equations. The first is a probit-type equation that predicts whether or not somebody responds. The second is a linear regression equation conditional on the individual providing a response. If it is assumed that the error terms of the two equations come from a bivariate normal distribution, which allows for a correlation between the two error terms and therefore the possibility of sample selection bias, the model can be estimated by **maximum likelihood estimation.**

In practice, the model is often estimated by a simpler two-step procedure. The first step is to estimate a probit equation for non-response and to save the **inverse Mills ratio**. The inverse Mills ratio is then added as an extra variable in the second stage regression of the outcome y on the set of explanatory variables. This second regression is estimated on the subsample of useable responses. Identification of the Heckit model can rely on finding some explanatory variables that enter the probit equation but do not enter the second stage regression. In the example given here, these are variables that influence whether somebody is willing to participate in the nurse visit, but do not influence their health outcome. In practice, it is often difficult to find such plausible identification restrictions, in which case the Heckit model is sometimes estimated with the same set of regressors in each equation. Then, identification relies on the non-linearity of the inverse Mills ratio. It is worth mentioning that a test of whether the coefficient of the inverse Mills ratio in the second stage regression is significantly different from zero also provides a test for the existence of sample selection bias. This test is given by the t-ratio associated with the inverse Mills ratio – a large value provides evidence of selection bias.

In practice, relying on identification by functional form can be problematic. A plot of the inverse Mills ratio shows that it is approximately linear for much of its range. The inverse Mills ratio is a function of the linear index $(x\beta)$ from the probit equation. This means that the range of the linear index, and hence of the explanatory variables in the probit equation, is important. It also means that the degree of censoring – in other words, the proportion of non-responders in the sample – is important, as this reduces the range of the observed values of the linear index. The performance of the sample selection model depends on the collinearity between the inverse Mills ratio and the explanatory variables in the regression equation. Collinearity is likely to be high if there are few or no regressors excluded from the second-stage regression, there is a high degree of non-response, there is low variability among the regressors in the probit equation or there is a large degree of unexplained variation in the probit equation. So it is advisable to check for collinearity. A simple way of doing this is to regress the inverse Mills ratio on the explanatory variables from the outcome equation and examine the goodness of fit of this equation. A high degree of goodness of fit indicates a high degree of collinearity.

An application to data from the nurse visit

One of the measures of physiological health collected at the nurse visit stage of HALS is the highest forced expiratory volume in one second ('hyfev'): a measure of lung capacity. Data on hyfev are only available for those who completed the nurse visit and, as we saw in Chapter 2, there is non-response at that stage of the survey. This gives us observations where there is item non-response on the outcome of interest but where the respondents' socio-economic characteristics were collected at the face-to-face interview (i.e. the x-values are not missing). In this case 2,258 observations are missing for hyfev out of the sample of 9,003.

To illustrate the sample selection model, we estimate a Heckit model for hyfev using the usual set of socioeconomic variables, to see if there is evidence of selection bias. Table 7.1 shows the **full-information maximum likelihood (FIML)** estimates of the model, based on estimating the joint model for both the selection equation and the outcome equation. The upper panel of results, labelled 'y', is the outcome equation for hyfev, the second panel, labelled 'select' is the probit equation for selection. Here the model is estimated without exclusion restrictions, so the same set of regressors appears in both equations. In this case the estimated correlation coefficient (ρ) is not statistically significant and the **likelihood ratio (LR) test** does not reject independence of the two error terms. Likelihood ratio tests are used to test hypotheses, in the form of restrictions on parameters, with **maximum likelihood estimators**. The LR statistic compares the value of the log-likelihood when estimation is unconstrained to the value when the parameters are restricted. Twice the difference between the log-likelihood values has a chi-squared distribution, which can be used to assess the statistical significance of the test statistic. The degrees of freedom for the statistic are given by the number of restrictions to be tested.

In this case the LR test suggests that selection bias is not a problem for the model estimated. However, a plot of the inverse Mills ratio (*see* Figure 7.1) shows that there is very little nonlinearity for the sample used here and identification of the model is likely to be tenuous. Notice the strong effects of gender and age in the model for hyfev (y). Subsequent analysis might split the sample by gender and refine the specification of the age effects, or alternatively include interactions between age and gender and, perhaps, between gender and other variables.

Table 7.1: Heckit model of fev

Heckman selection model (regression model with sample selection)		Number of obs = 9003

Heckman selection model
(regression model with sample selection)

Log likelihood = −10843.15

Number of obs = 9003
Censored obs = 2258
Uncensored obs = 6745
Wald chi2(25) = 8486.82
Prob > chi2 = 0.0000

	Coef.	Std. Err.	z	P > |z|	[95% Conf. Interval]	
y						
male	.8125755	.0184519	44.04	0.000	.7764105	.8487405
age	−.0310882	.0007944	−39.14	0.000	−.0326452	−.0295313
ethbawi	−.4314307	.0807154	−5.35	0.000	−.5896301	−.2732313
ethipb	−.6267204	.0636767	−9.84	0.000	−.7515244	−.5019164
ethothnw	−.369819	.0879738	−4.20	0.000	−.5422445	−.1973936
part	.013866	.0257336	0.54	0.590	−.036571	.064303
unemp	.0075395	.033918	0.22	0.824	−.0589387	.0740176
retd	−.1158967	.028611	−4.05	0.000	−.1719733	−.0598201
stdnt	−.0409793	.0723422	−0.57	0.571	−.1827674	.1008088
keephse	−.0602973	.0250754	−2.40	0.016	−.1094441	−.0111504
lsch14u	−.2316595	.0449365	−5.16	0.000	−.3197334	−.1435855
lsch14	−.1907123	.0260085	−7.33	0.000	−.241688	−.1397366
lsch15	−.0486662	.0202939	−2.40	0.016	−.0884415	−.0088908
lsch17	−.0126451	.0279633	−0.45	0.651	−.0674521	.042162
lsch18	.0699791	.0282967	2.47	0.013	.0145186	.1254396
lsch19	.0692228	.0631395	1.10	0.273	−.0545283	.1929739
regsc1s	.163703	.0339348	4.82	0.000	.097192	.230214
regsc2	.1136789	.0202273	5.62	0.000	.0740342	.1533237
regsc3n	.0494727	.0236284	2.09	0.036	.0031618	.0957835
regsc4	−.0711332	.0215751	−3.30	0.001	−.1134196	−.0288469
regsc5n	−.1600946	.0326568	−4.90	0.000	−.2241007	−.0960885
widow	−.0213705	.0301676	−0.71	0.479	−.0804979	.0377569
single	−.1191876	.0234896	−5.07	0.000	−.1652263	−.0731488
seprd	−.0698698	.0498066	−1.40	0.161	−.167489	.0277494
divorce	−.0558322	.0370699	−1.51	0.132	−.1284878	.0168235
_cons	3.795019	.0405287	93.64	0.000	3.715585	3.874454
select						
male	.232573	.035812	6.49	0.000	.1623827	.3027633
age	−.0059726	.0015541	−3.84	0.000	−.0090186	−.0029266
ethbawi	−.4546571	.1326604	−3.43	0.001	−.7146667	−.1946475
ethipb	−.2880392	.1173545	−2.45	0.014	−.5180497	−.0580286
ethothnw	−.2514401	.1658729	−1.52	0.130	−.576545	.0736648
part	.1789932	.0533689	3.35	0.001	.074392	.2835944
unemp	−.0333973	.0697933	−0.48	0.632	−.1701897	.1033952
retd	−.0328158	.0566798	−0.58	0.563	−.1439062	.0782746
stdnt	−.2451405	.139298	−1.76	0.078	−.5181597	.0278786
keephse	.0628335	.0509431	1.23	0.217	−.0370131	.1626801
lsch14u	−.0744573	.0864209	−0.86	0.389	−.2438392	.0949246
lsch14	−.0688098	.0523831	−1.31	0.189	−.1714789	.0338593
lsch15	−.019623	.0427149	−0.46	0.646	−.1033427	.0640967
lsch17	.0636893	.0592132	1.08	0.282	−.0523664	.1797451

Table 7.1: (Continued)

	Coef.	Std. Err.	z	P > |z|	[95% Conf. Interval]	
lsch18	.0295772	.0600879	0.49	0.623	−.0881929	.1473472
lsch19	.0128696	.13225	0.10	0.922	−.2463356	.2720749
regsc1s	.0953826	.0736921	1.29	0.196	−.0490512	.2398164
regsc2	.038184	.0422582	0.90	0.366	−.0446406	.1210086
regsc3n	−.1118837	.0468095	−2.39	0.017	−.2036287	−.0201387
regsc4	−.0910835	.042832	−2.13	0.033	−.1750328	−.0071343
regsc5n	−.1480804	.0625997	−2.37	0.018	−.2707735	−.0253872
widow	−.022733	.0562409	−0.40	0.686	−.1329631	.0874971
single	−.1842038	.0458182	−4.02	0.000	−.2740058	−.0944018
seprd	−.0990204	.0982883	−1.01	0.314	−.291662	.0936211
divorce	.0847648	.0789265	1.07	0.283	−.0699284	.2394579
_cons	.9301763	.0720145	12.92	0.000	.7890305	1.071322
/athrho	.2008323	.1100569	1.82	0.068	−.0148753	.4165399
/lnsigma	−.5383386	.0130823	−41.15	0.000	−.5639795	−.5126978
rho	.1981751	.1057346			−.0148742	.3940115
sigma	.5837172	.0076364			.5689405	.5988778
lambda	.1156782	.0628664			−.0075378	.2388942

LR test of indep. eqns. (rho = 0): chi2(1) = 1.65 Prob > chi2 = 0.1989

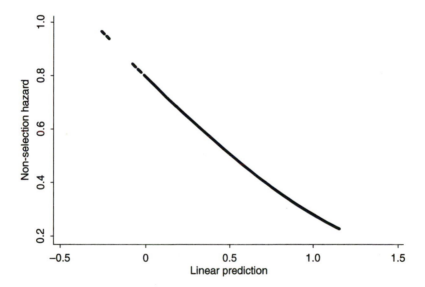

Figure 7.1: Inverse Mills ratio from fev application.

The results of the selection part of the model show that, on average and holding other factors constant, men and part-time workers are significantly more likely to have responded to the nurse visit. Older people, those from ethnic minorities, those who have never married and those from lower socioeconomic groups are less likely to have responded.

Appendix: Stata code for the sample selection model

The sample selection model (SSM/Heckman selection model/generalised tobit model) can be obtained using the **full information maximum likelihood estimator (FIML)**:

```
heckman yvar $xvars, select($xvars)
```

Alternatively, the Heckman two-step consistent estimates can be used, with an option to save the **inverse Mills ratio** as a new variable 'imr':

```
heckman yvar $xvars, select($xvars) twostep mills(imr)
```

Here the model is estimated without exclusion restrictions, so that the same set of x variables appears in the selection equation and the outcome equation. The shape of the inverse Mills ratio for the relevant range of the data can be plotted against the linear index:

```
probit regfag $xvars
predict yfp, xb
twoway scatter imr yfp
```

Also 'imr' can be regressed on the x variables to gauge the degree of collinearity:

```
regress imr $xvars
```

Chapter 8

Endogenous regressors: the evaluation problem revisited

The problem restated

Chapter 1 introduced an example of the evaluation problem: how to estimate the 'treatment effect' of ownership of private insurance on the use of healthcare. From a policy point of view it is of critical importance to know whether, and to what extent, an observed association between insurance and utilisation is due to selection effects or to a direct utilisation effect or both. If the observed insurance effect is entirely due to self-selection of those more likely to use healthcare, then private insurance coverage merely acts as a marker for such propensity and reducing private insurance options will not reduce the use of care. If, on the other hand, the insurance effect is mostly due to the utilisation effect of increased coverage, then the expansion or reduction of private insurance options will have an impact on use.

Therefore, a central question is whether access to private insurance encourages greater utilisation or not. This may be due to price effects ('moral hazard'), risk reduction effects, access effects or income-transfer effects. All these factors may encourage greater utilisation and they will be referred to collectively as the 'insurance effect' on utilisation. For example, in a system where private insurance provides supplementary cover alongside a universal public system that offers a basic package of services that are free at the point of use, the access effect may be the prime reason for increased utilisation among those with private cover.

Given the econometric methods discussed in Chapters 3 and 6, the specific example of an evaluation problem can now be formulated in terms of binary variables for whether an individual has private health insurance and whether they have used healthcare, for example by visiting a specialist. It is convenient and intuitive to describe the methods available to estimate the treatment effect of insurance on specialist visits under two broad headings: selection on observables and selection on unobservables.

Selection on observables

Those who receive the treatment (insurance) may differ systematically from those who do not receive the treatment (no insurance) in terms of their observable characteristics, so that confounding factors are non-randomly distributed over the treated and control individuals. These confounding factors may themselves be related to the use of healthcare. For example, those with insurance may be older and more affluent than those without insurance. Selection on observables approaches take account of these observable confounders.

Simple probit model

The simplest approach is to include the observable confounders in the regression model for the outcome of interest. So the baseline estimate of the insurance effect is given by the partial effect of private health insurance in a simple probit model for a visit to the specialist. As well as insurance coverage (y_1), the model for any specialist visit (y_2) conditions on a set of individual characteristics (x) by including them in the regression model. So:

$$P(y_{2i} = 1|y_{1i}, x_i) = \Phi(\gamma y_{1i} + \beta'x_i)$$

where $\Phi(.)$ is the standard normal distribution function. The **average treatment effect (ATE)** of insurance on specialist visits (the 'insurance effect') is computed by taking the sample mean of the **partial effect (PE)** for each individual observation. The partial effect is:

$$PE_i = \Delta P(y_{2i} = 1|y_{1i}, x_i)/\Delta y_{1i} = \Phi(\gamma + \beta'x_i) - \Phi(\beta'x_i).$$

The average treatment effect (ATE) is given by the mean across-the-sample observations:

$$ATE = \frac{1}{n}\sum_i \Delta P(y_{2i} = 1| y_{1i}, x_i)/\Delta y_{1i} = \frac{1}{n}\sum_i \{\Phi(\gamma + \beta'x_i) - \Phi(\beta'x_i)\}$$

As well as reporting the average effect, the availability of individual-specific partial effects allows us to explore heterogeneity in the effect across individuals, for example by displaying a histogram of the effects.

Inverse probability weighting (IPW)

The inverse probability weighted estimator is commonly used to deal with survey non-response and attrition (*see* Chapter 11). This approach is grounded in the notion of missing at random or ignorable non-response and relies on the assumption that, conditional on observed covariates, the probability of non-response does not vary systematically with the outcome of interest. The same concept can be applied to the estimation of treatment effects. This is motivated by the conceptual framework known as Rubin's Causal Model. In this framework each individual has two potential outcomes, the one that applies to their actual treatment (say, having insurance) and the other, counterfactual, outcome that would have occurred if they had received the alternative treatment (no insurance). The evaluation problem arises because only one of these potential outcomes can be observed for each individual. With a randomised experiment, with a 50:50 allocation rule, there would be an equal chance of observing either potential outcome. But if there is selection bias, making a particular individual more likely to be insured, then the potential outcome is 'over-represented' in the observed data.

Inverse probability weighting can correct for this 'unrepresentative' non-random sampling of potential outcomes by giving less weight to those individuals who have a high probability of their observed treatment, conditional on the set of observable covariates. These weights are then used in the computation of the average treatment effect. The IPW approach is valid if an ignorability condition holds: that the allocation to treatment is independent of the outcome of interest, conditional on the set of observables used to compute the weights.

Propensity score matching (PSM)

Matching also addresses the problem that in the observed data, confounding factors (matching variables) are non-randomly distributed over the treated and control individuals. But it does this without assuming a particular parametric model, such as a probit, for the outcome of interest. The idea is to match each treated individual with one or more controls who are comparable in terms of their observed characteristics. Rather than matching on an entire set of observable characteristics, the dimensions of the problem can be reduced by matching on the basis of their probability of receiving treatment, $P(y_{1i} = 1|x_i)$, known as the **propensity score**. With one-for-one matching of cases and controls those observations that are selected as controls effectively get a weight of one, while those that are not get a weight of zero. In practice, PSM estimators do not rely on exact matching and instead weight observations by their proximity, in terms of their propensity score.

In the application to estimating an insurance effect we could construct the propensity score using a probit model for insurance as a function of observable confounding factors. Then matching would use the predicted probability of having insurance. Treated (insured) individuals would be matched with non-treated (uninsured) individuals inversely weighted for the distance in terms of predicted propensities. More precisely, weights are typically constructed using some form of smoothed distance weighting.

In applying PSM methods it is important to check whether the treated and controls have common support: so, for each subset of values of the observables it is possible to find controls to match the treated cases. The quality of the matching can be assessed by computing the reduction of the **pseudo R-squareds** from regressions of insurance on the set of observables on the samples before and after matching. To evaluate the extent to which matching on propensity scores balances the distribution of the x-values between the insured and the uninsured group it is possible to compute the bias reduction due to matching for each of the x-values.

It should be noted that an important requirement of PSM is that the participation model used to construct the propensity score should include only variables that are unaffected by participation, or the anticipation of participation. This suggests that matching variables should be either time invariant characteristics or variables that are measured before participation in the treatment and that are not affected by anticipation of participation.

Selection on unobservables

The approaches described above rely on the assumption that, conditional on observables, there is no systematic (non-random/non-ignorable) variation in the allocation of treatments. This rules out idiosyncratic and unobservable individual characteristics that influence treatment (insurance) and are associated with the outcome (use). 'Selection on unobservables' estimators attempt to deal with this problem. These include **instrumental variable (IV)** and **Heckit** estimators, which are two-step approaches that rely on exploiting exogenous variation in the treatment variable that is independent of the outcome. For example, the IV approach searches for instruments: variables that are good predictors of participation in the treatment and that are independent of the outcome. Rather than pursuing these two-step approaches, here we concentrate on specifying a joint model of the treatment and outcome and estimating this structural model by **full information maximum likelihood (FIML)** estimation.

The FIML estimator for a recursive bivariate probit model

Here we can adopt a structural approach, in which the outcome equation includes the treatment variable as an endogenous regressor. This can be estimated by full information maximum likelihood estimation, based on FIML estimates of a recursive bivariate probit model. The first issue in specifying a structural model for insurance and specialist visits is how to specify a coherent econometric model that allows for the potential endogeneity of insurance. Coherency means that the model should be logically consistent, for example that the probabilities implied by the model should lie between 0 and 1 and add up to 1. Blundell and Smith's (1993) framework defines type I and type II specifications. In the type II model, actual insurance coverage (the binary variable) is assumed to influence healthcare use. In the type I model it is the latent index that influences use. The coherency conditions for the type II model imply that the model is only logically consistent when it is specified as a recursive system. In other words, the type II specification can only be coherent when the endogeneity of insurance stems from unobservable heterogeneity bias rather than a direct effect of the use of healthcare on having insurance.

In our application a type II specification makes more sense than a type I specification: we want to identify the impact of actually having private insurance on specialist visits rather than the impact of the propensity to have insurance. For this reason we could adopt a recursive model in which insurance coverage is assumed to influence the probability of a specialist visit; in this case the dummy variable for insurance coverage appears as a regressor in the equation for healthcare use. The insurance variable may be an endogenous regressor due to unobservable heterogeneity, such as an individual's level of risk or risk aversion, which has a direct influence on both their decision to take out insurance and their use of healthcare in the subsequent wave. This unobservable heterogeneity can be captured by using a **bivariate probit** specification and the model can be estimated using the standard estimation routines for the bivariate probit. The **partial effects** of insurance in this model can be computed from the marginal distribution for specialist visits, using the same formula as the univariate probit, but with the parameter estimates from the bivariate probit model.

It is only necessary to have variation in the set of exogenous regressors to avoid identification problems in this recursive bivariate probit model and exclusion restrictions are not required: this is often described as 'identification by functional form'. However, because identification by functional form relies heavily on the assumption of bivariate normality, it is common practice to impose exclusion restrictions to improve identification. The technical appendix provides more detail for the recursive bivariate probit model and shows how the FIML approach can be extended using quadrature, simulation estimation or mixture models.

Smoking and health revisited

As an application of the evaluation problem we apply the recursive bivariate probit model to the variables used in Chapter 6. The outcome is the binary measure of excellent or good self-assessed health ('sah') and the treatment is the binary indicator for current smokers ('regfag'). Unlike the model presented in Chapter 6, smoking is included as an endogenous regressor in the equation for health.

To set the scene Table 8.1 presents estimates from a simple probit equation that includes smoking as a regressor and the usual set of observables ('xvars'), but does not allow for selection on unobservables. The results are presented as coefficients, for comparability with Table 8.2 below. The coefficient of interest – on 'regfag' – is –0.283, showing a negative association between smoking and the probability of reporting good or excellent health. Note that the corresponding partial effect, computed using dprobit, is –0.098. This implies that the probability of reporting good or excellent health, evaluated at the means of the data, is 0.098 lower among smokers compared to non-smokers.

Table 8.1: Model of smoking and sah: simple probit

Probit estimates			Number of obs = 8998			
			LR chi2(26) = 459.93			
			Prob > chi2 = 0.0000			
Log likelihood = –5168.8942			Pseudo R2 = 0.0426			

sah	Coef.	Std. Err.	z	P > |z|	[95% Conf. Interval]	
regfag	–.2834219	.0307467	–9.22	0.000	–.3436842	–.2231596
male	.0379357	.0347104	1.09	0.274	–.0300954	.1059667
age	–.0023416	.0015505	–1.51	0.131	–.0053805	.0006973
ethbawi	–.3003068	.1347904	–2.23	0.026	–.5644912	–.0361224
ethipb	–.2703993	.1179187	–2.29	0.022	–.5015157	–.0392829
ethothnw	–.3090098	.165725	–1.86	0.062	–.6338249	.0158053
part	.1794459	.0533712	3.36	0.001	.0748401	.2840516
unemp	–.1109379	.0658615	–1.68	0.092	–.2400241	.0181484
retd	–.0619139	.0558293	–1.11	0.267	–.1713372	.0475095
stdnt	–.0020371	.1482554	–0.01	0.989	–.2926123	.2885381
keephse	–.0730751	.0502922	–1.45	0.146	–.171646	.0254958
lsch14u	–.2057873	.0848912	–2.42	0.015	–.3721709	–.0394037
lsch14	–.2078376	.0517547	–4.02	0.000	–.309275	–.1064002
lsch15	–.0607926	.0417539	–1.46	0.145	–.1426288	.0210436
lsch17	.0756232	.059379	1.27	0.203	–.0407575	.1920039
lsch18	.2489473	.0637648	3.90	0.000	.1239706	.3739241
lsch19	.0165733	.1320117	0.13	0.900	–.2421649	.2753115
regscls	.2355734	.075753	3.11	0.002	.0871002	.3840466
regsc2	.222422	.0421591	5.28	0.000	.1397918	.3050522
regsc3n	.0731073	.0464669	1.57	0.116	–.0179661	.1641807
regsc4	–.0866744	.0412053	–2.10	0.035	–.1674353	–.0059135
regsc5n	–.1894432	.0599798	–3.16	0.002	–.3070015	–.0718849
widow	–.1592316	.0554745	–2.87	0.004	–.2679596	–.0505035
single	–.1686212	.0453161	–3.72	0.000	–.2574392	–.0798032
seprd	–.2094371	.0953026	–2.20	0.028	–.3962267	–.0226475
divorce	–.1423799	.0737189	–1.93	0.053	–.2868662	.0021065
_cons	.8427513	.0729825	11.55	0.000	.6997081	.9857945

Table 8.2: Model of smoking and sah: recursive bivariate probit (sah equation only)

Seemingly unrelated bivariate probit	Number of obs = 8998
	Wald chi2(51) = 1021.75
Log likelihood = −10558.445	Prob > chi2 = 0.0000

	Coef.	Std. Err.	z	P > |z|	[95% Conf. Interval]	
sah						
regfag	−.612163	.4069364	−1.50	0.132	−1.409744	.1854177
male	.042915	.0350105	1.23	0.220	−.0257043	.1115344
age	−.0034022	.0019909	−1.71	0.087	−.0073043	.0004998
ethbawi	−.3319239	.1386194	−2.39	0.017	−.6036129	−.0602348
ethipb	−.2991636	.1216479	−2.46	0.014	−.537589	−.0607381
ethothnw	−.2829821	.168814	−1.68	0.094	−.6138514	.0478871
part	.1690912	.0551323	3.07	0.002	.0610339	.2771486
unemp	−.0599719	.0925363	−0.65	0.517	−.2413397	.121396
retd	−.0753073	.0576874	−1.31	0.192	−.1883725	.037758
stdnt	−.0332022	.1523305	−0.22	0.827	−.3317645	.2653602
keephse	−.0716603	.0501342	−1.43	0.153	−.1699215	.0266009
lsch14u	−.1823585	.0901028	−2.02	0.043	−.3589568	−.0057603
lsch14	−.1745779	.0673946	−2.59	0.010	−.3066688	−.042487
lsch15	−.027812	.0585759	−0.47	0.635	−.1426186	.0869946
lsch17	.0769114	.0590527	1.30	0.193	−.0388297	.1926525
lsch18	.2244963	.0710126	3.16	0.002	.0853141	.3636785
lsch19	.0155077	.1313448	0.12	0.906	−.2419233	.2729387
regscls	.1869534	.0971456	1.92	0.054	−.0034485	.3773554
regsc2	.1909239	.0589856	3.24	0.001	.0753142	.3065336
regsc3n	.0456185	.0578521	0.79	0.430	−.0677695	.1590065
regsc4	−.0802659	.0420466	−1.91	0.056	−.1626757	.0021439
regsc5n	−.1674007	.0669369	−2.50	0.012	−.2985945	−.0362068
widow	−.15941	.0552586	−2.88	0.004	−.2677149	−.0511051
single	−.1682737	.045176	−3.72	0.000	−.2568171	−.0797304
seprd	−.1571888	.116693	−1.35	0.178	−.3859029	.0715253
divorce	−.0934628	.0964646	−0.97	0.333	−.28253	.0956045
_cons	.9858715	.1801555	5.47	0.000	.6327732	1.33897
/athrho	.202791	.2591514	0.78	0.434	−.3051364	.7107185
rho	.2000562	.2487796			−.2960061	.6111272

Likelihood-ratio test of rho=0:   chi2(1) = .502653   Prob > chi2 = 0.4783

Variable	Obs	Mean	Std. Dev.	Min	Max
ate	9003	−.2102048	.0243423	−.2404574	0
Variable	Obs	Mean	Std. Dev.	Min	Max
atet	2956	−.2091503	.0278615	−.2453971	−.0935849

Table 8.2 presents the results of the recursive bivariate probit model, which explicitly models the selection on unobservables. In this case the model is estimated without exclusion restrictions, relying on functional form to identify the model. In the full Stata output the first panel of results is for the sah equation and the second is for the regfag equation, but for brevity Table 8.2

only presents the former. The coefficient on regfag increases in absolute size to –0.612, although the standard error on the coefficient increases as well, and the LR test for $\rho = 0$ does not reject the null hypothesis. However, the estimated average treatment effect (ATE) is –0.21 as is the estimated average treatment effect on the treated (ATET). These estimates are shown at the foot of Table 8.2. The ATET is the average effect of the treatment on the outcome for those who would adopt the treatment. In this case it measures the impact of smoking on health among those who become smokers, rather than for the population as a whole. This finding suggests that selection bias may be causing an underestimate of the effect of smoking on health in the simple probit equation and deserves further attention. For example, 'frailer' individuals who have a tendency to suffer from respiratory problems may be more likely to quit smoking, and be observed as non-smokers in the dataset, but also be more likely to report poor health. One option would be to search for plausible exclusion restrictions to impose (effectively searching for good 'instruments' for smoking).

Appendix: Stata code for estimating treatment effects

Linear outcome and binary treatment

This chapter has concentrated on dealing with binary outcomes and treatments. Here we begin by presenting some Stata code for the more straightforward case of a linear (continuous) outcome and a binary treatment. An example from HALS is to use a measure of lung capacity (forced expiratory volume in one second) as the outcome and cigarette smoking as the treatment:

```
replace yvar2=hyfev1
replace yvar1=regfag
```

Selection on observables

The simplest of the 'selection on observables approaches' is to run a linear regression of 'hyfev1' on 'regfag', conditioning on the observed covariates x:

```
regress yvar2 yvar1 $xvars
```

Inverse probability weights can be calculated using a **probit model** for the allocation into treatment ('yvar1'). The formula for the weights depends on each individual's value of 'yvar1', those with a high probability of their observed treatment are given less weight. Here the weights are used in a regression model for 'yvar2':

```
probit yvar1 $xvars
predict pi, p
gen ipw = 1
replace ipw=1/pi if yvar1 == 1
replace ipw=1/(1-pi) if yvar1 == 0
summ ipw
regress yvar2 yvar1 [pweight=ipw]
```

Stata provides numerous options for implementing propensity score matching, along with other forms of matching. The simplest default option is:

```
psmatch2 yvar1 $xvars, out(yvar2)
```

Selection on unobservables

The Heckman treatment effects model for a linear outcome can be implemented as follows, assuming a different set of variables z (including some 'instruments') are used to predict treatment:

```
regr yvar2 yvar1 $xvars
treatreg yvar2 $xvars, treat(yvar1 = $zvars) twostep
treatreg yvar2 $xvars, treat(yvar1 = $zvars)
```

While the linear **instrumental variables (IV)** estimator is:

```
ivreg yvar2 $xvars (yvar1 = $zvars)
```

Binary outcome and binary treatment

Here we concentrate on the code for estimating the recursive bivariate probit model. The treatment is current smoking 'regfag' and the binary outcome is self-assessed health, 'sah':

```
replace yvar2=sah
```

For comparison we begin with the standard univariate probit model, estimated using 'probit' and 'dprobit':

```
probit yvar2 yvar1 $xvars
dprobit yvar2 yvar1 $xvars
```

Then we estimate the recursive model, with the treatment, 'yvar1', appearing as a regressor in the outcome equation for 'yvar2'. The predicted values of the linear index from each equation are saved so they can be used to calculate **partial effects**:

```
biprobit (yvar2=yvar1 $xvars) (yvar1=$xvars)
predict yf1, xb1
predict yf2, xb2
```

The average treatment effect (ATE) of smoking on health can be computed using the standard formula for the partial effect on the marginal probability p(sah = 1):

```
scalar b1_pbt=_b[yvar1]
gen ate=0
replace ate=norm(yf1+b1_pbt)-norm(yf1) if yvar1==0
replace ate=norm(yf1)-norm(yf1-b1_pbt) if yvar1==1
summ ate
hist ate
```

Also the average treatment effect of the treated (ATET) can be computed using the partial effect on the conditional probability p(sah=1|regfag=1):

```
scalar rho=_b[athrho:_cons]
gen atet=0
replace atet=norm((yf1+b1_pbt-rho*yf2)/(1-rho^2)^0.5) -
norm((yf1-rho*yf2)/(1-rho^2)^0.5) if yvar1==0
replace atet= norm((yf1-rho*yf2)/(1-rho^2)^0.5) -
norm((yf1-b1_pbt-rho*yf2)/(1-rho^2)^0.5) if yvar1==1
summ atet if yvar1==1
hist atet if yvar1==1
```

Chapter 9

Count data regression

Methods

The measure of self-assessed health used in previous chapters is an example of an ordered categorical variable. For convenience this was coded as y = 0, 1, 2..., but these numerical values are arbitrary. Count data regression applies to dependent variables coded in the same way, where the values are meaningful in themselves; in other words, where the dependent variable represents a count of events. Common examples in health economics include measures of healthcare utilisation, such as the number of times an individual visits their GP during a given period, or the number of prescriptions dispensed to an individual. Count data regression is appropriate when the dependent variable is a non-negative integer valued count, y = 0, 1, 2..., where y is measured in natural units on a fixed scale. Typically, count data regression is applied when the distribution of the dependent variable is skewed. The data will usually contain a large proportion of zero observations, for example those who make no use of healthcare during the survey period, as well as a long right-hand tail of individuals who make particularly heavy use of healthcare.

The basic statistical model for count data assumes that the probability of an event occurring (λ) during a brief period of time is constant and proportional to the duration of time. λ is known as the intensity of the process. The starting point for count data regression is the Poisson process. To turn this into an econometric model where the outcome y depends on a set of explanatory variables x, it is usually assumed that $\lambda = \exp(x\beta)$. The exponential function is used to ensure that the intensity of the process, which can also be interpreted as the mean number of events, given x, is always positive.

An important feature of the **Poisson regression** model is the **equi-dispersion** property. This means that the mean of y, given x, equals the variance of y, given x. For the Poisson model to be appropriate, this assumption should be reflected in the observed data. In practice, the distribution of many of the variables of interest to health economists, such as measures of healthcare utilisation, display **over-dispersion**. In other words, the mean of the variable is smaller than the variance of the variable. Many of the recent developments of count data regression have aimed to relax this restrictive feature of the Poisson model and to introduce models that allow for **under-** or **over-dispersion** in the data.

Two basic approaches are used to estimate count data regressions. Once the probability of a given count is specified, it is possible to use **maximum likelihood estimation**. This uses the fully specified probability distribution and maximises a sample likelihood function. The maximum likelihood approach builds in the assumption that the conditional mean of the dependent variable has the exponential form described above. It also builds in other features of the distribution, such as the equi-dispersion property of the Poisson model. If the conditional mean specification is correct, but there is under- or over-dispersion in the data, then maximum likelihood estimates of the standard errors of the regression coefficients and the t-tests will be biased. However, count data regressions have a convenient property that, as long as the conditional mean is correctly specified, maximum likelihood estimates of the βs will be **consistent**. This is true even if other assumptions about the distribution, such as equi-dispersion, are invalid. This useful property is known as **pseudo maximum likelihood estimation (PMLE)**. In this case the model should be estimated with robust standard errors.

The definition of the intensity of the process tells us that the mean of y, given x, is an exponential function of a linear index in the explanatory variables. This has the form of a non-linear regression function and means that count data models can also be estimated using a nonlinear least squares approach. In particular, many recent applications of count data models use the **generalised method of moments (GMM)** estimator. This approach only rests on the assumption that the conditional mean is correctly specified, rather than the full probability distribution, and is therefore more robust than maximum likelihood estimation.

An application to cigarette smoking

Table 9.1 shows an example of the **Poisson regression** model. The dependent variable is the number of cigarettes smoked per day by respondents to the HALS. Respondents are asked to report the actual number of cigarettes, and the variable can be interpreted as a count. The model estimates the number of cigarettes smoked as a function of the usual list of explanatory variables. Table 9.1 reports the coefficients, standard errors and implied z-ratios for each of the variables. Recall that the coefficients relate to the intensity of the process, which is a non-linear function of the x-values. So the βs are not measured in the original units of the count data and inferences about the impact of a particular variable on the actual number of counts have to be made by retransforming the coefficient estimates. However, we can use the coefficients to analyse the qualitative impacts of the variables. So, for example, the results show a strong socioeconomic gradient in the number of cigarettes smoked, with those in professional and managerial occupations having negative coefficients and the variables for semi-skilled and unskilled occupations having positive coefficients.

Inferences about quantitative effects can be made by calculating the marginal effect for a continuous explanatory variable, say x_k, which is given by the formula:

$$\partial E(y|x)/\partial x_k = \beta_k \exp(x\beta), \tag{7}$$

while the formula for the average effect of a binary variable is:

$$E(y|x_k = 1) - E(y|x_k = 0) = \exp(x\beta|x_k = 1) - \exp(x\beta|x_k = 0). \tag{8}$$

As with binary choice models, it is clear that these marginal and average effects depend on the values of the other explanatory variables. Again, standard practice is to evaluate these at the mean of the other x-values, but estimates can be calculated for every individual in the sample. Average effects for the discrete regressors and marginal effects for the continuous regressors are given in Table 9.2, along with the mean value of each regressor.

Table 9.1: Poisson regression for cigarettes per day

Poisson regression

Number of obs = 8881
LR chi2(27) = 11237.48
Prob > chi2 = 0.0000
Log likelihood = −60409.332
Pseudo R2 = 0.0851

yvar	Coef.	Std. Err.	z	P > |z|	[95% Conf. Interval]	
male	.2084821	.0117404	17.76	0.000	.1854714	.2314928
age	−.0105308	.000819	−12.86	0.000	−.012136	−.0089255
age2	−.0839595	.0028981	−28.97	0.000	−.0896397	−.0782793
age3	−.0487911	.0117997	−4.13	0.000	−.0719181	−.0256641
ethbawi	−.8141589	.0616801	−13.20	0.000	−.9350497	−.6932681
ethipb	−.5500904	.049943	−11.01	0.000	−.6479769	−.4522039
ethothnw	−.0063454	.0584604	−0.11	0.914	−.1209257	.1082348
part	−.1064703	.0170825	−6.23	0.000	−.1399513	−.0729893
unemp	.2894559	.017382	16.65	0.000	.2553877	.323524
retd	−.0306639	.0231153	−1.33	0.185	−.0759691	.0146413
stdnt	−.3541118	.0680278	−5.21	0.000	−.4874439	−.2207797
keephse	−.0282476	.0161667	−1.75	0.081	−.0599337	.0034384
lsch14u	.4431014	.0303888	14.58	0.000	.3835405	.5026623
lsch14	.332869	.0182712	18.22	0.000	.297058	.3686799
lsch15	.2827287	.0134964	20.95	0.000	.2562763	.3091812
lsch17	−.0124955	.0204422	−0.61	0.541	−.0525614	.0275704
lsch18	−.4090868	.0239678	−17.07	0.000	−.4560629	−.3621107
lsch19	−.280291	.0527058	−5.32	0.000	−.3835926	−.1769895
regsc1s	−.6155476	.0305427	−20.15	0.000	−.6754102	−.555685
regsc2	−.2591576	.0139296	−18.60	0.000	−.2864591	−.231856
regsc3n	−.2963375	.0161676	−18.33	0.000	−.3280254	−.2646496
regsc4	.0402827	.012723	3.17	0.002	.015346	.0652194
regsc5n	.1951064	.0175924	11.09	0.000	.160626	.2295869
widow	.1033594	.0225812	4.58	0.000	.059101	.1476178
single	.0455864	.015946	2.86	0.004	.0143329	.0768399
seprd	.5266067	.024033	21.91	0.000	.4795029	.5737105
divorce	.3720886	.0195796	19.00	0.000	.3337133	.410464
_cons	1.698063	.0173809	97.70	0.000	1.663997	1.732129

The results in Tables 9.1 and 9.2 are estimated by maximum likelihood, assuming that the Poisson distribution is appropriate for the data on the number of cigarettes smoked. In fact, this is unlikely to be valid. In particular, there is a very high proportion of zeros in the observed data. Around 70% of individuals were not current smokers at the time of the survey. Among other things, this means that the conditional mean of the data does not equal the conditional variance and leads us to look for specifications that allow for **over-dispersion** and what are known as '**excess zeros**'. In other words, the data exhibit a higher frequency of zero observations than would be predicted by the simple Poisson model.

One possible explanation for over-dispersion and excess zeros is additional individual heterogeneity beyond differences that can be summarised by the observed explanatory variables. Mullahy (1997) emphasises that the presence of

Table 9.2: Partial effects for Poisson regression for cigarettes per day

Marginal effects after poisson
    y = predicted number of events (predict)
      = 4.6479522

variable	dy/dx	X
male*	.984229	.433960
age	−.0489466	.841797
age2	−.3902397	3.13685
age3	−.2267785	.241804
ethbawi*	−2.611021	.010472
ethipb*	−1.982213	.014413
ethothnw*	−.0294013	.007319
part*	−.4755526	.121608
unemp*	1.537752	.050332
retd*	−.1413172	.221371
stdnt*	−1.391851	.011823
keephse*	−.1299703	.140187
lsch14u*	2.549311	.036933
lsch15*	1.406401	.271704
lsch17*	−.0577811	.088616
lsch18*	−1.618129	.088616
lsch19*	−1.140367	.013287
regsc1s*	−2.212712	.056976
regsc2*	−1.124598	.224186
regsc3n*	−1.242925	.141088
regsc4*	.1897727	.167098
regsc5n*	.989656	.060241
widow	.4804094	.085801
single	.2118833	.170701
seprd	2.447643	.021619
divorce	1.72945	.037496

(*) dy/dx is for discrete change of dummy variable from 0 to 1

excess zeros in count data can be seen as a strict implication of unobservable heterogeneity. Up to now individual differences only enter the model through differences in the x variables. If there are additional unobservable differences across individuals, these could be added as an extra unobservable variable or error term. The effect of adding this further heterogeneity is to spread out the distribution of the count variable, meaning that more observations are shifted to the tails of the distribution, so that we would expect to observe more zero values and more high values than would be predicted by the simple Poisson model.

The most commonly applied model that allows for additional unobservable heterogeneity is the negative binomial or **negbin model**, which allows for over-dispersion by assuming that the individual error term comes from a particular probability distribution (the **gamma distribution**). By assuming the gamma distribution it is possible to write down a new probability function for y and hence to estimate the model by **maximum likelihood estimation**. The negbin model

Table 9.3: Negative binomial model for cigarettes per day

Negative binomial regression

Number of obs = 8881
LR chi2(27) = 263.52
Prob > chi2 = 0.0000
Pseudo R2 = 0.0074

Log likelihood = −17697.843

yvar	Coef.	Std. Err.	z	P > |z|	[95% Conf. Interval]	
male	.239186	.0758291	3.15	0.002	.0905638	.3878083
age	−.0085022	.0050999	−1.67	0.095	−.0184979	.0014935
age2	−.0813607	.0186917	−4.35	0.000	−.1179958	−.0447256
age3	−.0419942	.0614688	−0.68	0.494	−.1624708	.0784824
ethbawi	−.7740075	.3144606	−2.46	0.014	−1.390339	−.157676
ethipb	−.6184399	.2669483	−2.32	0.021	−1.141649	−.0952308
ethothnw	−.0107198	.3696925	−0.03	0.977	−.7353038	.7138643
part	−.1351946	.1108069	−1.22	0.222	−.3523721	.0819829
unemp	.2971866	.1482682	2.00	0.045	.0065862	.587787
retd	−.054419	.1367701	−0.40	0.691	−.3224835	.2136454
stdnt	−.4090891	.3164427	−1.29	0.196	−1.029305	.2111273
keephse	−.0458872	.1086378	−0.42	0.673	−.2588134	.167039
lsch14u	.3767383	.1958954	1.92	0.054	−.0072097	.7606862
lsch14	.2157437	.1177754	1.83	0.067	−.0150919	.4465793
lsch15	.2576711	.0947917	2.72	0.007	.0718827	.4434594
lsch17	.0042482	.125851	0.03	0.973	−.2424153	.2509116
lsch18	−.393168	.1300719	−3.02	0.003	−.6481042	−.1382317
lsch19	−.3720131	.2830083	−1.31	0.189	−.9266991	.1826729
regsc1s	−.5046795	.1601508	−3.15	0.002	−.8185692	−.1907897
regsc2	−.2879881	.0893091	−3.22	0.001	−.4630307	−.1129455
regsc3n	−.3526389	.1020198	−3.46	0.001	−.5525941	−.1526838
regsc4	−.0033635	.0924934	−0.04	0.971	−.1846472	.1779203
regsc5n	.1644896	.1372828	1.20	0.231	−.1045797	.4335589
widow	.1867993	.1330337	1.40	0.160	−.0739419	.4475405
single	.0685149	.1077326	0.64	0.525	−.142637	.2796669
seprd	.5293877	.2140531	2.47	0.013	.1098514	.9489241
divorce	.4541375	.164771	2.76	0.006	.1311923	.7770826
_cons	1.729985	.1163724	14.87	0.000	1.501899	1.958071
/lnalpha	2.111045	.0227965			2.066364	2.155725
alpha	8.256861	.1882273			7.896063	8.634146

Likelihood ratio test of alpha = 0: chibar2(01) = 8.5e+04 Prob>=chibar2 = 0.000

is more flexible and relaxes the equi-dispersion property of the Poisson model. Two special cases of the negbin model are typically estimated in practice: one in which the variance of y is proportional to the mean of y, and the other in which the variance is a quadratic function of the mean. An attractive feature of the negbin model is that it nests the Poisson model as a special case and this can be tested using a conventional t-test on the coefficient that reflects over-dispersion. The negbin model has been applied extensively in studies of healthcare utilisation (*see* Jones 2000 for a review of this literature).

Table 9.3 shows estimates of a negbin model for the number of cigarettes smoked. The conditional mean function for the negbin model is still an exponential function of the explanatory variables and the coefficients should be interpreted in just the same way as the Poisson model. The additional parameter α estimates the degree of over-dispersion in the data. By default Stata estimates the negbin2 version of the model in which the variance is a quadratic function of the mean. This parameter is large (8.257) and highly significant. In this example there is strong evidence to reject the Poisson specification as a special case of the negbin. The qualitative results for the negbin model are broadly comparable with those of the Poisson model. So, for example, we again see a socioeconomic gradient in the level of smoking, and there are some small changes in the magnitudes of the coefficients and substantial changes in the standard errors and t-ratios.

Recall that our dependent variable is heavily influenced by a large proportion of zero observations – around 70% of the sample. It is likely that much of the distinction between smokers and non-smokers is now being picked up by the estimate of over-dispersion. However, like the Poisson model, the negbin model assumes that there is a single process underlying all of the observed values of the dependent variable, whether y equals 0 or is greater than 0. Other recent developments of count data regression have been based on the idea that there is something special about the zero observations and that they are not just a reflection of over-dispersion. This makes a qualitative distinction between participants and non-participants, for example between those who use health care and those who do not, or between smokers and non-smokers. One example of this kind of approach is so-called **zero-inflated models**. These are an example of **mixture models**. They take a standard count data model such as the Poisson or negative binomial and add extra weight to the probability of observing a zero value. This probability can be interpreted as a splitting mechanism that divides individuals into non-users, with a probability q, and potential users with probability 1 – q. The probability q may be a function of a set of explanatory variables. So, in the zero-inflated model the probability of observing zero is made up of the probability of someone being a non-user plus the probability that they are a potential user, multiplied by the probability of observing a zero under the standard count data model.

Tables 9.4 and 9.5 show estimates of the zero-inflated negative binomial regression for the number of cigarettes smoked (again the estimated model is a negbin2 specification). The first set of results (Table 9.4) assumes the splitting mechanism is just a constant. The second (Table 9.5) allows explanatory variables to influence the splitting mechanism. These show evidence of a split between non-smokers and potential smokers, and also that this split is influenced by observable explanatory variables – many of the variables that appear in the splitting equation, labelled *inflate* in Table 9.5, are statistically significant. Notice also that there are now substantial differences in both the sign and the size of the regression coefficients for the negbin regression model compared to the specification that did not allow for zero inflation. For example, the negbin results in Table 9.5 no longer show such a clear socioeconomic gradient in the level of smoking. This suggests that the earlier results were largely driven by the distinction between smokers and non-smokers, and that effectively the count data regressions were acting like binary choice models, explaining whether someone smokes rather than how much they smoke.

The zero-inflated specification separates out the binary choice of whether to smoke or not from the number of cigarettes smoked, given that someone is a smoker. Another way of dealing with this distinction between participants and non-participants is to use a so-called **hurdle** or two-part specification. This

Table 9.4: Zero-inflated negbin model for cigarettes per day: I

Zero-inflated negative binomial regression			Number of obs = 8881			
			Nonzero obs = 2914			
			Zero obs = 5967			
Inflation model = logit			LR chi2(27) = 291.89			
Log likelihood = −15749.16			Prob > chi2 = 0.0000			

yvar	Coef.	Std. Err.	z	P>|z|	[95% Conf. Interval]	
yvar						
male	.165783	.024712	6.71	0.000	.1173485	.2142176
age	−.002588	.001747	−1.48	0.138	−.006012	.000836
age2	−.0421808	.006039	−6.98	0.000	−.0540171	−.0303445
age3	.0558082	.0240881	2.32	0.021	.0085965	.1030199
ethbawi	−.4568471	.1134162	−4.03	0.000	−.6791388	−.2345553
ethipb	−.2997162	.0999778	−3.00	0.003	−.4956691	−.1037632
ethothnw	−.228455	.1164398	−1.96	0.050	−.4566728	−.0002371
part	−.0354273	.0357876	−0.99	0.322	−.1055697	.0347152
unemp	−.0225922	.037748	−0.60	0.550	−.096577	.0513926
retd	−.1184293	.0466222	−2.54	0.011	−.2098071	−.0270515
stdnt	−.1078132	.1348282	−0.80	0.424	−.3720717	.1564453
keephse	−.0310741	.0338928	−0.92	0.359	−.0975028	.0353547
lsch14u	.1087141	.065943	1.65	0.099	−.0205318	.2379601
lsch14	.0246182	.0393796	0.63	0.532	−.0525645	.1018009
lsch15	.0458843	.0293772	1.56	0.118	−.011694	.1034626
lsch17	−.0176921	.0432019	−0.41	0.682	−.1023662	.066982
lsch18	−.0963355	.0500321	−1.93	0.054	−.1943966	.0017257
lsch19	−.2110032	.1064913	−1.98	0.048	−.4197223	−.0022841
regsc1s	.0646949	.0667196	0.97	0.332	−.066073	.1954628
regsc2	.033021	.0300546	1.10	0.272	−.0258849	.0919268
regsc3n	−.0642388	.0339188	−1.89	0.058	−.1307185	.0022409
regsc4	−.0116592	.0271075	−0.43	0.667	−.064789	.0414706
regsc5n	.0404697	.0379354	1.07	0.286	−.0338823	.1148218
widow	.0449928	.0464207	0.97	0.332	−.04599	.1359757
single	.0033871	.0336483	0.10	0.920	−.0625624	.0693366
seprd	.1752159	.0547423	3.20	0.001	.067923	.2825088
divorce	.0554193	.0429662	1.29	0.197	−.0287929	.1396315
_cons	2.808045	.0372049	75.48	0.000	2.735124	2.880965
inflate						
_cons	.7144212	.0226187	31.59	0.000	.6700895	.758753
/lnalpha	−1.527933	.035427	−43.13	0.000	−1.597369	−1.458498
alpha	.2169836	.0076871			.2024284	.2325854

Table 9.5: Zero-inflated negbin model for cigarettes per day: II

. zinb yvar $xvars if wave==1, inflate($xvars _cons);

Zero-inflated negative binomial regression					Number of obs = 8881	

Nonzero obs = 2914

Zero obs = 5967

Inflation model = logit   LR chi2(27) = 290.19

Log likelihood = −15419.93   Prob > chi2 = 0.0000

yvar	Coef.	Std. Err.	z	P > |z|	[95% Conf. Interval]	
yvar						
male	.1651176	.0246702	6.69	0.000	.1167649	.2134702
age	−.0026078	.0017422	−1.50	0.134	−.0060225	.0008069
age2	−.0419216	.0060272	−6.96	0.000	−.0537346	−.0301085
age3	.0575564	.0238905	2.41	0.016	.0107319	.1043809
ethbawi	−.45416	.1130194	−4.02	0.000	−.6756739	−.2326462
ethipb	−.2975508	.09964	−2.99	0.003	−.4928415	−.1022601
ethothnw	−.2293836	.1163446	−1.97	0.049	−.4574148	−.0013524
part	−.0356723	.0357427	−1.00	0.318	−.1057266	.0343821
unemp	−.0229508	.0377367	−0.61	0.543	−.0969134	.0510119
retd	−.1196494	.0465099	−2.57	0.010	−.2108071	−.0284918
stdnt	−.1044109	.1341013	−0.78	0.436	−.3672447	.1584229
keephse	−.0312997	.033858	−0.92	0.355	−.0976602	.0350608
lsch14u	.1071627	.0657906	1.63	0.103	−.0217845	.2361099
lsch14	.0241309	.0393051	0.61	0.539	−.0529058	.1011675
lsch15	.0456296	.0293469	1.55	0.120	−.0118893	.1031485
lsch17	−.0178212	.0431329	−0.41	0.679	−.1023601	.0667177
lsch18	−.0951733	.0498875	−1.91	0.056	−.192951	.0026044
lsch19	−.209386	.106156	−1.97	0.049	−.4174478	−.0013241
regsc1s	.0660621	.0664783	0.99	0.320	−.064233	.1963573
regsc2	.0334974	.0300076	1.12	0.264	−.0253164	.0923112
regsc3n	−.0634174	.0338604	−1.87	0.061	−.1297825	.0029477
regsc4	−.0115948	.0270846	−0.43	0.669	−.0646796	.04149
regsc5n	.0403628	.0379119	1.06	0.287	−.0339431	.1146687
widow	.0443472	.0462971	0.96	0.338	−.0463935	.1350879
single	.0035342	.0336015	0.11	0.916	−.0623235	.0693919
seprd	.1748827	.0547107	3.20	0.001	.0676517	.2821136
divorce	.0549495	.042945	1.28	0.201	−.0292211	.1391201
_cons	2.808213	.0371605	75.57	0.000	2.735379	2.881046
inflate						
male	−.0942922	.0580971	−1.62	0.105	−.2081603	.019576
age	.0127342	.0040913	3.11	0.002	.0047154	.0207531
age2	.0620747	.0142394	4.36	0.000	.034166	.0899834
age3	.1243065	.0547056	2.27	0.023	.0170856	.2315275
ethbawi	.5341702	.2412783	2.21	0.027	.0612734	1.007067
ethipb	.5119719	.2181043	2.35	0.019	.0844953	.9394484
ethothnw	−.3434212	.2744485	−1.25	0.211	−.8813304	.194488
part	.1044786	.0846668	1.23	0.217	−.0614652	.2704224
unemp	−.6145025	.1056705	−5.82	0.000	−.8216129	−.407392
retd	−.1293913	.1099201	−1.18	0.239	−.3448308	.0860481
stdnt	.3740523	.2761051	1.35	0.175	−.1671037	.9152083

Table 9.5: (Continued)

yvar	Coef.	Std. Err.	z	P>|z|	[95% Conf. Interval]	
keephse	−.0189792	.0813432	−0.23	0.816	−.178409	.1404506
lsch14u	−.4630782	.1533632	−3.02	0.003	−.7636645	−.1624919
lsch14	−.4331438	.0911224	−4.75	0.000	−.6117405	−.2545472
lsch15	−.3681723	.0696687	−5.28	0.000	−.5047204	−.2316243
lsch17	−.0140726	.096944	−0.15	0.885	−.2040793	.1759341
lsch18	.429907	.1066641	4.03	0.000	.2208492	.6389647
lsch19	.1317406	.2291932	0.57	0.565	−.3174699	.5809511
regscl1s	.869616	.1368796	6.35	0.000	.6013368	1.137895
regsc2	.4539897	.0690051	6.58	0.000	.3187422	.5892372
regsc3n	.3767895	.0772583	4.88	0.000	.2253661	.5282129
regsc4	−.0716924	.0671394	−1.07	0.286	−.2032833	.0598985
regsc5n	−.2585987	.099083	−2.61	0.009	−.4527977	−.0643997
widow	−.1072686	.1042935	−1.03	0.304	−.3116801	.0971429
single	−.0822875	.0817644	−1.01	0.314	−.2425427	.0779677
seprd	−.6518891	.1533489	−4.25	0.000	−.9524475	−.3513308
divorce	−.6073318	.117501	−5.17	0.000	−.8376295	−.3770341
_cons	.697431	.0869027	8.03	0.000	.5271048	.8677571
/lnalpha	−1.530275	.0353395	−43.30	0.000	−1.599539	−1.461011
alpha	.2164762	.0076502			.2019897	.2320017

assumes that the participation decision and the positive values of the count data are generated by two separate probability functions. In some applications, the participation decision is modelled using a standard binary choice model such as the logit or probit. In others, a count data specification such as the Poisson or negbin model is used, with a dependent variable that can take values of either 0 or 1. Then a standard count data regression is applied to the subsample of participants, allowing for the fact that the count data is truncated at zero.

When faced with count data that exhibit **over-dispersion** and a large proportion of zero observations, analysts are faced with a choice of two types of specification: those that emphasise the role of unobservable heterogeneity, such as the negbin model; and those that emphasise the special role of zero observations, such as zero-inflated or hurdle models. Applications of zero-inflated or hurdle models often make the probability of participation a function of explanatory variables, as interest lies in the types of factor that distinguish users and non-users of healthcare, or smokers and non-smokers. Applications of the negbin model often treat over-dispersion as a fixed parameter and do not allow it to be a function of the explanatory variables. This may bias the comparison in favour of zero-inflated and hurdle models. The negbin model also relies on a specific functional form for the unobservable heterogeneity. Recent work in the health economics literature has advocated a more robust and flexible approach, which treats unobservable heterogeneity in a non-parametric way: the **finite mixture** approach to model healthcare utilisation. In this approach, the unobservable heterogeneity is treated as a discrete random variable where each category of the variable represents an unobservable 'type' of individual. So, for example, with a two-point mixture there would be two types, such as 'healthy' and 'ill' individuals. These two values are known as points of support.

In the finite mixture approach, the probability of an individual belonging to one of these types is estimated along with the other parameters of the model. Deb and Trivedi (1997) apply finite mixture models with two and three points of support for data on the demand for medical care among individuals aged 66 and over in the 1987 US medical care expenditure survey. Demand is measured by six different indicators of annual healthcare utilisation and the finite mixture model is compared to hurdle and zero-inflated specifications. The negbin models with two points of support are preferred on the basis of various statistical criteria. Deb and Trivedi interpret the points of support as two latent populations of 'healthy' and 'ill' individuals, reflecting unobservable differences in frailty across the population.

Appendix: Stata code for count data regression

The count data regression models are applied to 'fagday', the number of cigarettes smoked per day:

```
replace yvar=fagday
```

Poisson regression

The starting point is the Poisson regression model. Predictions are saved for both the fitted values of the nonlinear regression function, $\exp(x\beta)$ and for the linear index, $x\beta$:

```
poisson yvar $xvars
* predict exp(xb)
predict fitted, n
predict yf, xb
```

Partial effects of the regressors on the actual number of cigarettes smoked need to take account of the nonlinearity of the regression function, $\exp(x\beta)$. Here we compute the average effect for 'unemp':

```
scalar bunemp=_b[unemp]
gen ae_unemp=0
replace ae_unemp=exp(yf+bunemp)-exp(yf) if unemp==0
replace ae_unemp=exp(yf)-exp(yf-bunemp) if unemp==1
summ ae_unemp
hist ae_unemp
```

One way of assessing the performance of the model is to tabulate the actual and fitted values of y against each other. To do this, the fitted values are rounded to the nearest integer value:

```
replace fitted=round(fitted)
tab fitted yvar
```

The RESET test for the Poisson model follows the usual format:

```
gen yf2=yf^2
quietly poisson yvar $xvars yf2
test yf2
```

To exploit the pseudo maximum likelihood (PML) property of Poisson regression the model can be estimated using robust standard errors:

```
poisson yvar $xvars, robust
```

The negbin model

To relax the **equi-dispersion** property that is implicit in the Poisson model we can run a negative binomial (**negbin**) regression and recalculate **partial effects** and the fitted values:

```
nbreg yvar $xvars
predict yf, xb
predict fitted
*PARTIAL EFFECTS
scalar bunemp=_b[unemp]
gen ae_unemp=0
replace ae_unemp=exp(yf+bunemp)-exp(yf) if unemp==0
replace ae_unemp=exp(yf)-exp(yf-bunemp) if unemp==1
summ ae_unemp
hist ae_unemp
scalar drop bunemp
drop ae_unemp
replace fitted=round(fitted)
tab fitted yvar
```

By default, Stata estimates the negbin2 version of the model in which the variance is a quadratic function of the mean. The alternative negbin1 specification, in which it is a linear function, can be obtained by using the subcommand dispersion(constant). A more general specification allows the over-dispersion to be a function of the x variables as well as the conditional mean:

```
gnbreg yvar $xvars, lna($xvars)
predict fitted
replace fitted=round(fitted)
tab fitted yvar
```

Zero-inflated models

The Poisson, negbin and generalised negbin models all assume the same mean function, $\exp(x\beta)$. This may not be flexible enough to model a dependent variable with excess zeros. One alternative is the **zero-inflated model** that adds an additional probability of observing a zero. The simplest form of the zero-inflated Poisson (ZIP) model treats this probability as a constant:

```
zip yvar $xvars, inflate(_cons)
predict fitted
predict yf
replace fitted=round(fitted)
tab fitted yvar
```

Computation of the partial effects needs to take account of the change in the mean function in the ZIP model:

```
scalar bunemp=_b[unemp]
scalar qi=_b[inflate:_cons]
scalar qi=exp(qi)/(1+exp(qi))
scalar list qi
gen ae_unemp=0
replace ae_unemp=(1-qi)*(exp(yf+bunemp)-exp(yf)) if unemp==0
replace ae_unemp=(1-qi)*(exp(yf)-exp(yf-bunemp)) if unemp==1
summ ae_unemp
hist ae_unemp
```

A more flexible version of the ZIP allows the zero-inflation probability q to depend on the regressors. This model can be difficult to estimate in practice and estimates may not converge:

```
zip yvar $xvars, inflate($xvars _cons)
predict pi, p
predict fitted
replace fitted=round(fitted)
tab fitted yvar
```

Similar syntax applies for the zero-inflated negbin model:

```
zinb yvar $xvars, inflate(_cons)
predict fitted
replace fitted=round(fitted)
tab fitted yvar
zinb yvar $xvars, inflate($xvars|_cons)
predict fitted
replace fitted=round(fitted)
tab fitted yvar
```

Hurdle models

A common alternative to the zero-inflated model is the hurdle model. The first stage of the **hurdle model** is often estimated as a standard logit model:

```
replace yvar1=regfag
logit yvar1 $xvars
```

Followed by truncated regressions (either Poisson or negbin) at the second stage:

```
ztp yvar $xvars
ztnb yvar $xvars
```

Chapter 10

Duration analysis

Duration data

The previous section discussed count data models, where the dependent variable is the number of events occurring over a period of time, for example the number of GP visits over the previous month. A closely related topic is duration analysis. Here, the focus is on the time elapsed before an event occurs, rather than on the number of events. So, for example, duration could measure the number of years that someone lives from birth; or it could measure a patient's length of stay after admission to hospital; or it could measure the number of years that someone smoked cigarettes.

Once again, the HALS can be used to provide a useful illustration of the application of duration analysis. Forster and Jones (2001) used duration analysis to explore two aspects of smoking: the decisions to start and to quit. Here, there are two measures of duration: the age at which somebody starts smoking cigarettes and the number of years that they smoke once they have started. By analysing these two variables we can learn about the impact of individual characteristics on the probability of starting and the probability of quitting smoking. Recall that the original HALS data were collected in 1984–85. The survey included information that allows individuals to be divided into those who were regular smokers at the time of the survey, those who had been regular smokers but had quit by the time of the survey and those who had never smoked prior to the survey.

The current and ex-smokers in the survey were asked how old they were when they started to smoke cigarettes. This is self-reported retrospective data and so may be prone to problems of measurement error, such as recall bias. Recall bias occurs when respondents have difficulty recalling events from their past, it includes phenomena such as 'telescoping' of events and 'heaping' of observations at round numbers.

For those who had started smoking at some time prior to the survey, we observe the actual value of duration and their age when they started smoking. For those individuals who had not smoked prior to the survey, there is a problem of censoring. In other words, all we know is that they had not started smoking prior to the date of the interview. It is possible that some of these individuals will go on to start smoking at a later age. All we know is that their age of starting is at least as great as their age at the time of the survey, and for this reason we refer to them as **right censored** observations. So for these individuals we can use the probability that their true duration is greater than the censored value – in this case, their age at the time of the HALS. Standard models of duration data are built on the assumption that eventually everyone will 'fail'. In this application, this would mean that eventually all individuals will start smoking. This is unlikely to be plausible in the case of smoking and, as we shall see below, it is possible to relax the specification to allow some individuals to remain non-smokers.

For those who become smokers the second measure of duration is the number of years that they smoke. This helps us to analyse the probability of quitting. This new variable can be defined by taking the individuals' ages at the time of the interview and subtracting the ages at which they started smoking. For those individuals who had already quit smoking prior to the survey, the number of years since they quit should also be subtracted. Once again, there is a problem of **right censoring**. For those individuals who had quit prior to the survey, we observe a complete spell from the time they start to the time they quit smoking. For those individuals who were still current smokers at the time of the survey, all we know is the age that they started and the fact that they are still smoking in 1984–85. For these individuals we can only estimate the probability that they have been smokers for at least that many years.

The HALS data provide us with a third measure of duration. The survey respondents were linked with the NHS Central Register of Deaths, which provides information on survival rates. For respondents who had died by June 2005 (the latest release of the deaths data), the survey provides information on their age and cause of death taken from death certificates. This third measure of duration is an individual's lifespan in years, with the origin defined as an individual's birth and the duration measured up to their age at death. Once again, there is a problem of **right censoring**. For those individuals who died between the collection of the HALS data in 1984 and the collection of the deaths data in 2005, we observe a complete spell. The majority of the original HALS respondents were still alive in 2005, and these represent right censored observations. But the deaths data raise a further issue, the problem of **left truncation**. The natural origin for the measure of lifespan is an individual's birth. However, the HALS was designed as a representative random sample of the living population in 1984. To be included in the survey, an individual must have survived at least to their age at the time of HALS. An individual who was born and died prior to HALS is a form of missing data. For each age group the probability of surviving to the time of the survey may vary systematically across different types of individuals. This creates a source of bias – the problem of left truncation. To deal with this, the duration models need to be adapted to incorporate the probability that an individual survives at least to their age at the time of HALS.

Survival analysis

Analysis of models of survival or duration revolves around the notion of a **hazard function** h(t). This measures the probability that someone fails at time t, given that they have survived up to that point. It can be written as:

$$h(t) = f(t)/S(t), \qquad (9)$$

where the two components on the right-hand side are the probability density function (f(t)), the probability of failing at time t and the survival function (S(t)), which is the probability that someone survives to at least time t. In estimating duration models, the density function is used for uncensored observations, where we observe their actual time of failure, and the survival function is used for censored observations where we only know they have survived at least to time t.

Parametric models of duration assume particular functional forms for f(t) and S(t) and therefore for the hazard function h(t). A common example is the **Weibull model**. The hazard function for the Weibull model takes the form:

$$h(t) = hpt^{p-1} \cdot \exp(x\beta), \qquad (10)$$

where h and p are parameters to be estimated. This develops the kind of regression model we have seen in previous chapters in that it is not just a function of the explanatory variables x but also of duration itself (t). The first term on the right-hand side of equation (10), hpt^{p-1}, is known as the baseline hazard. This defines the relationship between the hazard of failure and the duration (t). The shape of the baseline hazard allows us to estimate how the hazard function changes with time. In the Weibull model, the parameter p is known as the shape parameter. The hazard function is increasing for $p > 1$, showing increasing duration dependence, while it is decreasing for $p < 1$, showing decreasing duration dependence. Duration dependence may be of interest in itself. For example, we may want to learn whether the probability of someone receiving a job offer increases or decreases the longer they have been unemployed. In addition to learning about duration dependence, duration analysis allows us to estimate the impact of individual characteristics (the x-values) on the probability of failure. These are captured by the second term in equation (10), $\exp(x\beta)$, which leads to proportional shifts in the baseline hazard for individuals with different characteristics (x).

Parametric models rely on fully specifying the baseline hazard function. The chosen functional form may not be valid and it is particularly vulnerable to problems caused by unobservable heterogeneity across individuals. A more flexible approach is to use a semi-parametric model. The best-known example is the **Cox proportional hazard model**. This leaves the baseline hazard unspecified, treated as an unknown function of time. Because the method does not require specification of the baseline hazard, it is more robust than parametric approaches. In order to implement the method, the duration data are converted into a rank ordering of individuals according to their level of duration, t. Because this throws away information on the actual value of t, the method is less efficient than a parametric approach.

Analysis of the age of starting smoking is more complicated. As mentioned earlier, standard duration models assume that eventually everyone fails – in this case everyone would eventually start smoking. This seems to be an implausible assumption, and models based on the assumption do not do a good job of fitting the observed data. An alternative is to use a so-called **split population model**. This augments the standard duration analysis by adding a splitting mechanism analogous to the zero-inflated models of count data. So, for example, a probit specification could be added to model the probability that somebody will eventually start smoking. When this splitting mechanism is added to the duration model, it does a far better job of explaining the observed data on age of starting than models that omit a splitting mechanism (*see* Forster and Jones 2001).

As with count data, dealing with unobservable heterogeneity is a particular preoccupation in the literature on duration models. The existence of unobservable heterogeneity will bias estimates of duration dependence. For example, consider the case where there are two types of people: 'frail' individuals who have a high (but constant) hazard rate and 'strong' individuals who have a low (but constant) hazard rate. The two groups may be equally mixed in the population to begin with, but over time the frailer individuals will tend to die first, leading to an unequal mix. As time passes the proportion of frail individuals will decrease and the overall hazard will decrease. If it is not possible to control for the heterogeneity between the two types of individual, this will give the appearance of decreasing duration dependence. Unobservable heterogeneity can be dealt with by adding an extra error term to the model. Like count data models, this can be dealt with parametrically by assuming a particular functional form for the distribution of the error term. Alternatively, a non-parametric approach can be adopted, using the **finite mixture model**. This assumes that the unobservable error term has a discrete distribution characterised by a set of mass points, where the value of these mass points and the probabilities attached to them are estimated as part of maximum likelihood estimation.

An application to the HALS deaths data

The measure of survival time used in this application is each individual's lifespan. The entry date is the individual's date of birth and the exit date is June 2005, the time of the latest release of the HALS deaths data. Lifespan is left truncated, as the duration is only observed for those individuals who survived up to the HALS1 inter-view data, so the left truncation variable is age at HALS1. Those individuals who are still alive at June 2005 have incomplete spells and are treated as censored observa-tions. Table 10.1 reports descriptive evidence from the 'stsum' and 'stdes' commands for survival data. These show that the first quartile of survival time is 71 years, the median is 80 and the upper quartile is 87. They confim that the data only contain one record per subject and that the mean time of entry (age at HALS1) is 46 and the mean time of exit is 64. The latter includes all of the incomplete spells – those still alive in June 2005. There are 2,415 cases who had died by June 2005.

Table 10.1: Descriptive analysis of duration data for lifespan

| | incidence | | no. of | Survival time | | |
	time at risk	rate	subjects	25%	50%	75%
total	157982.2999	.0152865	8987	71.3	80.2	87.5

failure _d: death
analysis time _t: lifespan
id: serno

| | | | per subject | | | |
Category	total	mean	min	median	max
no. of subjects	8987				
no. of records	8987	1	1	1	1
(first) entry time	46.39813	18	44	98	
(final) exit time	63.97711	20.8	63	111	
subjects with gap	0				
time on gap if gap	0	.	.	.	.
time at risk	157982.3	17.57898	.0999985	20	21
failures	2415	.2687215	0	0	1

Before moving to the survival regressions, Figures 10.1 to 10.3 show the non-parametric estimates of the survival and hazard functions. These are based on the **Kaplan-Meier** estimator, which is a widely used non-paramet-ric estimator of survival functions. In Figure 10.1, the survival function remains fairly flat (with a high probability of survival) until the mid-60s age range. It then drops off rapidly, approaching zero as the age range reaches the late 90s. This pattern is reflected in the shape of the Kaplan-Meier estimate of the hazard function (Figure 10.2) and **Nelson-Aalen** estimate of the cumulative hazard function (Figure 10.3). The hazard is smooth and monotonically increasing. It remains flat until around age 60 and then increases quite dramatically as the risk of death rises with age. The dip in the hazard function at the extreme right of the age range is an artefact of the sparsity of data for the very elderly in HALS.

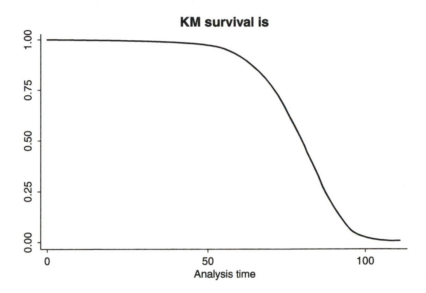

Figure 10.1: Kaplan-Meier survival curve for lifespan.

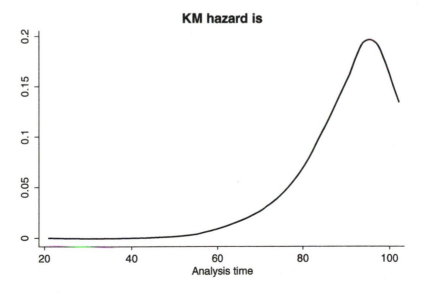

Figure 10.2: Kaplan-Meier hazard function for lifespan.

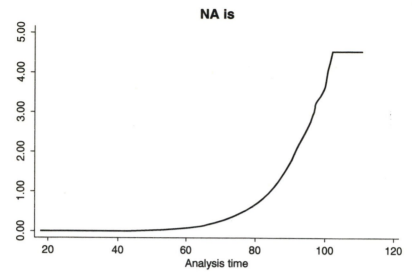

Figure 10.3: Nelson-Aalen cumulative hazard for lifespan.

We move now to the survival regressions that model the hazard as a function of a reduced set of our usual set of covariates. Table 10.2 presents the **Cox proportional hazard model** of lifespan. The coefficients are reported in the form of $\exp(\beta)$ and should be intepreted as upwards (>1) or downwards (<1) parallel shifts in the baseline hazard function. The results show some evidence of a gradient by education: those who left school later always have a lower probability (hazard) of death. The same applies to the social class gradient where the higher social classes have a lower hazard.

Table 10.2: Cox proportional hazard model of lifespan

Cox regression — Breslow method for ties
No. of subjects = 8987
No. of failures = 2415
Time at risk = 157982.2999

Number of obs = 8987

LR chi2(14) = 92.29
Prob > chi2 = 0.0000

Log likelihood = −17083.313

_t	Haz. Ratio	Std. Err.	z	P > |z|	[95% Conf. Interval]	
ethbawi	.6784805	.2576319	−1.02	0.307	.3223444	1.428087
ethipb	.6719269	.2143383	−1.25	0.213	.3595811	1.255588
ethothnw	1.084525	.3644599	0.24	0.809	.5612925	2.095512
lsch14u	1.195328	.1177616	1.81	0.070	.9854351	1.449926
lsch14	1.281497	.097581	3.26	0.001	1.103829	1.487761
lsch15	1.118036	.0968666	1.29	0.198	.9434257	1.324963
lsch17	1.223654	.129452	1.91	0.056	.9945091	1.505595
lsch18	.8518063	.1169974	−1.17	0.243	.6507685	1.114949
lsch19	.7203218	.2150499	−1.10	0.272	.4012387	1.293154
regscls	.6872238	.0832998	−3.09	0.002	.541904	.8715134
regsc2	.7801928	.0472086	−4.10	0.000	.6929417	.8784301
regsc3n	.8665275	.058551	−2.12	0.034	.7590439	.9892311
regsc4	1.05013	.0592246	0.87	0.386	.9402373	1.172867
regsc5n	1.062766	.085488	0.76	0.449	.9077535	1.24425

The model in Table 10.3 uses a parametric baseline hazard, in this case the **Weibull model**. Like Table 10.2 the results are presented in proportional hazard format and can be compared directly to those for the Cox model (which leaves the baseline hazard unspecified). It is clear that the estimates are very similar for both models. The estimate of the duration dependence parameter, p, is 7.382 showing strong positive duration dependence, as we would expect from the non-parametric plot of the hazard function. This is reflected in the plot of the fitted survival (Figure 10.4), hazard (Figure 10.5) and cumulative hazard (Figure 10.6) functions for the Weibull model, which are comparable to the nonparametric estimates.

Table 10.4 presents estimates for the same **Weibull model**, shown in accelerated time to failure format. This reformulation of the model can be interpreted as a regression of the x variables on the logarithm of lifespan. So the estimated coefficients should be interpreted in terms of changes in the logarithm of lifespan ($\ln(T)$). A positive sign means increased lifespan and a negative sign reduced lifespan for individuals with a particular characteristic. So while Table 10.3 presents results for $\exp(\beta)$, the coefficients in Table 10.4 give $-\ln\{\exp(\beta)\}/p$. To take the indicator for belonging to a professional occupation (*regsc1s*) as an example: in Table 10.3 the coefficient for this variable is 0.686, which is less than 1, meaning that the hazard of dying at a given age is

Table 10.3: Weibull regression for lifespan: proportional hazard form

Weibull regression — log relative-hazard form
No. of subjects = 8987
No. of failures = 2415
Time at risk = 157982.2999

Number of obs = 8987

LR chi2(14) = 96.01
Prob > chi2 = 0.0000

Log likelihood = 434.01297

_t	Haz. Ratio	Std. Err.	z	P > |z|	[95% Conf. Interval]	
ethbawi	.6712817	.2548562	−1.05	0.294	.3189635	1.412761
ethipb	.6625369	.2112575	−1.29	0.197	.3546457	1.237729
ethothnw	1.064585	.3577026	0.19	0.852	.5510295	2.056769
lsch14u	1.203339	.1180313	1.89	0.059	.9928797	1.458409
lsch14	1.248995	.0939584	2.96	0.003	1.077773	1.447419
lsch15	1.084224	.0929884	0.94	0.346	.9164647	1.282691
lsch17	1.211292	.1279005	1.82	0.069	.9848508	1.489798
lsch18	.8200914	.1124925	−1.45	0.148	.6267616	1.073055
lsch19	.7150631	.2133734	−1.12	0.261	.398426	1.283338
regsc1s	.6858299	.0829851	−3.12	0.002	.54103	.8693836
regsc2	.7709139	.0466587	−4.30	0.000	.6846803	.8680084
regsc3n	.8681134	.0586014	−2.10	0.036	.7605307	.9909146
regsc4	1.0534	.059375	0.92	0.356	.9432254	1.176445
regsc5n	1.066581	.0856728	0.80	0.422	.9112161	1.248436
/ln_p	1.999071	.0183589	108.89	0.000	1.963088	2.035054
p	7.382196	.135529			7.121287	7.652665
1/p	.135461	.0024869			.1306734	.1404241

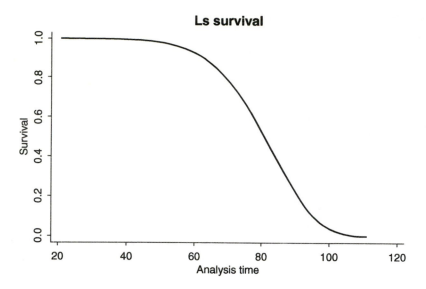

Figure 10.4: Weibull survival curve for lifespan.

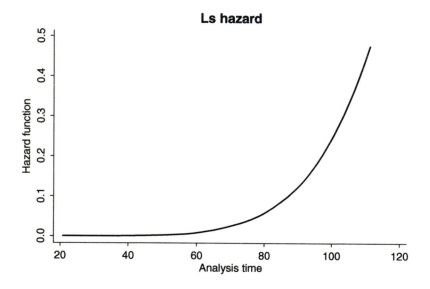

Figure 10.5: Weibull hazard function for lifespan.

lower for professional people than for the reference individual (with a skilled manual occupation). In Table 10.4 the coefficient is transformed to the time to failure scale and the estimate is 0.051 (= −ln(0.686)/7.382). This means that the log(lifespan) of professional people is estimated to be 0.051 longer on average than of those in skilled manual occupations; 0.051 on the log scale translates to just over a year of lifespan.

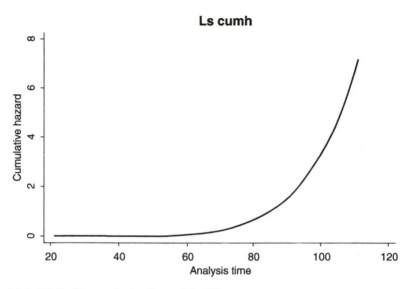

Ls cumh

Figure 10.6: Weibull cumulative hazard for lifespan.

Table 10.4: Weibull regression for lifespan: accelerated failure-time form

Weibull regression — accelerated failure-time form
No. of subjects = 8987   Number of obs = 8987
No. of failures = 2415
Time at risk = 157982.2999

LR chi2(14) = 96.01
Log likelihood = 434.01297   Prob > chi2 = 0.0000

_t	Coef.	Std. Err.	z	P > |z|	[95% Conf. Interval]	
ethbawi	.0539902	.0514705	1.05	0.294	−.04689	.1548705
ethipb	.0557665	.0432359	1.29	0.197	−.0289744	.1405073
ethothnw	−.0084778	.045513	−0.19	0.852	−.0976816	.080726
lsch14u	−.0250739	.0134062	−1.87	0.061	−.0513495	.0012017
lsch14	−.0301183	.0103201	−2.92	0.004	−.0503454	−.0098913
lsch15	−.010954	.011606	−0.94	0.345	−.0337013	.0117934
lsch17	−.0259662	.0143376	−1.81	0.070	−.0540674	.002135
lsch18	.0268673	.0185832	1.45	0.148	−.0095551	.0632897
lsch19	.0454315	.0404221	1.12	0.261	−.0337943	.1246573
regsc1s	.0510858	.0163761	3.12	0.002	.0189894	.0831823
regsc2	.0352441	.0081924	4.30	0.000	.0191872	.0513009
regsc3n	.0191586	.0091305	2.10	0.036	.0012631	.0370542
regsc4	−.0070471	.0076359	−0.92	0.356	−.0220132	.0079189
regsc5n	−.0087316	.0108853	−0.80	0.422	−.0300664	.0126032
_cons	4.439699	.0101855	435.89	0.000	4.419736	4.459662
/ln_p	1.999071	.0183589	108.89	0.000	1.963088	2.035054
p	7.382196	.135529			7.121287	7.652665
1/p	.135461	.0024869			.1306734	.1404241

Appendix: Stata code for duration analysis

The measure of survival time used in the application is each individual's lifespan. The entry date is the individual's date of birth and the exit date is June 2005, the time of the latest release of the deaths data. Lifespan is **left truncated**, as the duration is only observed for those individuals who survived up to the HALS1 interview data, so the left truncation variable is age at HALS1. Those individuals who are still alive at June 2005 have incomplete spells and are treated as **right censored** observations. These features of the data are encoded in the 'stset' command:

```
stset lifespan, failure(death) id(serno) time0(age)
```

Once this has been specified the duration variable 'lifespan' can be summarised:

```
stsum
stdes
```

Before proceeding to the estimation of survival regressions it is important to explore nonparametric plots of the survival and hazard functions. **Nelson-Aalen** and **Kaplan-Meier** estimates can be computed and the plots saved to files for subsequent use:

```
sts graph, na title('NA ls') saving(lsNA, replace)
sts graph, hazard  title('KM hazard ls') saving(lsHkm, replace)
sts graph, title('KM Survival ls') saving(lsKMsurv, replace)
```

The first regression model to be estimated is the **Cox proportional hazard model**, which leaves the baseline hazard unspecified. This uses a reduced set of regressors that capture ethnic group, education and social class, defined by the global '$xls':

```
stcox $xls
```

The parametric **Weibull model** can be estimated in comparable proportional hazard format:

```
streg $xls, d(weibull) nolog
```

Or it can be estimated using the accelerated time to failure version:

```
streg $xls, d(weibull) nolog time
```

This is followed up by commands to plot and save the fitted survival, cumulative hazard and hazard functions:

```
stcurve, survival title('Ls survival') saving(lssurv, replace)
stcurve, cumh title('Ls cumh') saving(lscumh, replace)
stcurve, hazard title('Ls hazard') saving(lshaz, replace)
```

Chapter 11

Panel data models

Linear models

With the exception of duration analysis, all of the models described so far have been applied to a single cross-section survey, where each individual is observed only once. With **panel data** a longitudinal element is added to the data and there are repeated measurements for each individual observation. Panel data are closely related to multilevel data where observations are grouped within organisations or geographic areas: for example, a survey of patients, within specialties, within hospitals. Multilevel models have a similar structure to models for panel data and are not discussed here (*see* Further reading).

Recall that the original HALS cross-section study was repeated seven years later in 1991–92. Rather than drawing a new random sample of individuals, the original HALS respondents were revisited and asked to complete the same face-to-face interview, nurse visit and postal questionnaire as in the original study. So, for each variable in the survey, and for each individual respondent, we observe two values. With only two waves, HALS is an example of a so-called 'short' panel where the number of individuals, n, is far greater than the number of waves, T. Longitudinal data add a new dimension to the analysis and allow researchers to explore the dynamics of individual behaviour. They also provide more scope for dealing with individual heterogeneity.

Consider a standard linear regression model in which there are repeated measurements (t = 1, ... ,T) for a sample of n individuals (i = 1, ... ,n):

$$y_{it} = x_{it}\beta + \alpha_i + \varepsilon_{it}. \tag{11}$$

Here the dependent variable y is observed for individual, i, in each of the waves, t. Similarly, the explanatory variables x are observed at each wave. Some of these variables will be time varying (for example, an individual's income at different points of time). Others may be fixed or time invariant (such as an individual's gender or ethnic background). In practice, with the kind of short panels discussed here, the regressors may also include a set of dummy variables for each wave of the panel (with one wave omitted for the reference period) in order to capture time effects. The error term of the regression equation (11) has been split into two components (this is known as an **error components model**). The first term, α_i, is an individual-specific unobservable effect – the unobserved characteristics of the individual i that remain constant over time. The second term, ε_{it}, is a random error term representing idiosyncratic shocks that vary over time. Typically, it is assumed that α_i and ε_{it} are uncorrelated with each other. The critical issue for the estimation of panel data models is whether the individual effects α_i are correlated with the observed regressors x. Failure to account for correlation between α_i and x in estimating the panel data regression model leads to inconsistent estimates of the slope coefficients, β.

The presence of a common individual effect means that the values of the dependent variable for each individual will tend to cluster together. This clustering can be allowed for using the **generalised least squares estimator (GLS)**, which allows for the fact that an error term for a particular individual will be correlated over the waves of the panel. However, use of the GLS estimator assumes that the individual effect is uncorrelated with the explanatory variables x. This problem can be dealt with by using deviations to sweep the unobservable individual effect out of the equation. One way of doing this is to adopt a **fixed effects** approach and take mean deviations, measuring each variable as the deviation from within-individual mean of the variables. Alternatively the variables can be measured as first differences (by subtracting the value in period t − 1 from the value in period t). Because the individual effect is assumed to be constant over time, taking deviations eliminates α from the equation. Applying the standard least squares estimator to the transformed variables gives the covariance or within-groups estimator of β, which is consistent even when the individual effect is correlated with the explanatory variables. However, for this estimator to work in practice, there must be sufficient within-individual variability in the dependent variable and the explanatory variables. The estimator will tend not to work well in a short panel (where t is small) and where there is not much variation within groups. These problems go away when the group size is large, in other words when t is large. In that case the **GLS** or **random effects** estimator can be shown to be equivalent to the within-groups or **fixed effects** estimator.

The **random effects** and **fixed effects** estimators for the linear panel data model are illustrated using data on the number of cigarettes smoked per day for the subsample of smokers in the HALS data. Table 11.1 shows the random effects GLS regression and Table 11.2 shows the fixed effects within-groups regression. The models are estimated using the two waves of the HALS data. As some individuals who took part in the first survey did not respond to, or could not be traced for, the second survey, the models are estimated on the **unbalanced panel**, using all available observations on the dependent variable. This means that more data are included for individuals at wave 1 than for wave 2.

Table 11.1: Linear random effects model for cigarettes per day (GLS)

Random-effects GLS regression Number of obs = 4342
Group variable (i) : serno   Number of groups = 3062
R-sq: within = 0.0535   Obs per group: min = 1
  between = 0.0966   avg = 1.4
  overall = 0.0911   max = 2
Random effects u_i ~ Gaussian Wald chi2(27) = 396.57
corr(u_i, X) = 0 (assumed)   Prob > chi2 = 0.0000

yvar	Coef.	Std. Err.	z	P > |z|	[95% Conf. Interval]	
male	2.898659	.3396536	8.53	0.000	2.23295	3.564368
age	−.0304106	.0215193	−1.41	0.158	−.0725876	.0117664
age2	−.6439257	.0761712	−8.45	0.000	−.7932185	−.4946329
age3	.5998144	.2800377	2.14	0.032	.0509507	1.148678
ethbawi	−5.859856	1.596165	−3.67	0.000	−8.988283	−2.73143
ethipb	−4.795425	1.43272	−3.35	0.001	−7.603505	−1.987344
ethothnw	−3.686484	1.686421	−2.19	0.029	−6.991809	−.3811602
part	−.8124215	.415153	−1.96	0.050	−1.626106	.0012634
unemp	−1.013121	.4948661	−2.05	0.041	−1.983041	−.0432012
retd	−1.520195	.5347246	−2.84	0.004	−2.568235	−.4721536
stdnt	.183426	1.542036	0.12	0.905	−2.838909	3.205761
keephse	−.4214062	.4262893	−0.99	0.323	−1.256918	.4141055
lsch14u	2.081061	.975074	2.13	0.033	.1699509	3.992171
lsch14	.5854126	.558657	1.05	0.295	−.5095351	1.68036
lsch15	1.140985	.4170894	2.74	0.006	.3235052	1.958466
lsch17	.235464	.6325691	0.37	0.710	−1.004349	1.475277
lsch18	−.9055674	.7327179	−1.24	0.216	−2.341668	.5305333
lsch19	−2.69433	1.582058	−1.70	0.089	−5.795106	.406446
regsc1s	.4088833	.8065552	0.51	0.612	−1.171936	1.989702
regsc2	.1463989	.3887129	0.38	0.706	−.6154643	.9082621
regsc3n	−.8087709	.4412171	−1.83	0.067	−1.673541	.0559988
regsc4	−.0969798	.3478152	−0.28	0.780	−.7786852	.5847255
regsc5n	.7526405	.4842886	1.55	0.120	−.1965477	1.701829
widow	1.030657	.59798	1.72	0.085	−.1413624	2.202676
single	.017102	.4613643	0.04	0.970	−.8871553	.9213594
seprd	3.444529	.6674898	5.16	0.000	2.136273	4.752785
divorce	.7209378	.5041313	1.43	0.153	−.2671413	1.709017
_cons	16.18108	.48061	33.67	0.000	15.23911	17.12306

sigma_u 6.5221676
sigma_e 5.4933769
rho   .58499852 (fraction of variance due to u_i)

Table 11.2: Linear fixed effects model for cigarettes per day

Fixed-effects (within) regression	Number of obs = 4342	
Group variable (i) : serno	Number of groups = 3062	
R-sq: within = 0.0648	Obs per group: min = 1	
between = 0.0341	avg = 1.4	
overall = 0.0362	max = 2	
	$F(17,1263)= 5.15$	
corr(u_i, Xb) = −0.0951	Prob > F = 0.0000	

yvar	Coef.	Std. Err.	t	P > |t|	[95% Conf. Interval]	
male	(dropped)					
age	−.0413616	.0449158	−0.92	0.357	−.1294795	.0467562
age2	−.8270015	.1331349	−6.21	0.000	−1.088191	−.5658115
age3	.2895262	.4886271	0.59	0.554	−.669084	1.248136
ethbawi	(dropped)					
ethipb	(dropped)					
ethothnw	(dropped)					
part	−.3915503	.5977959	−0.65	0.513	−1.564333	.781232
unemp	−3.055652	.787098	−3.88	0.000	−4.599815	−1.511488
retd	−.6765088	.7617225	−0.89	0.375	−2.170889	.8178718
stdnt	1.680867	2.361335	0.71	0.477	−2.951703	6.313437
keephse	−.4300261	.6682942	−0.64	0.520	−1.741115	.881063
lsch14u	(dropped)					
lsch14	(dropped)					
lsch15	(dropped)					
lsch17	(dropped)					
lsch18	(dropped)					
lsch19	(dropped)					
regscls	.2942756	1.379834	0.21	0.831	−2.412744	3.001295
regsc2	.2913165	.7241938	0.40	0.688	−1.129439	1.712072
regsc3n	.4087132	.8046426	0.51	0.612	−1.16987	1.987296
regsc4	−.1300566	.5771256	−0.23	0.822	−1.262287	1.002174
regsc5n	1.211408	.8220318	1.47	0.141	−.40129	2.824106
widow	1.832758	1.188608	1.54	0.123	−.4991061	4.164622
single	.3852976	1.038784	0.37	0.711	−1.652634	2.42323
seprd	3.020071	.9732749	3.10	0.002	1.110658	4.929485
divorce	.1297901	.8413171	0.15	0.877	−1.520743	1.780323
_cons	18.23225	.4476278	40.73	0.000	17.35407	19.11042

sigma_u	8.4461331	
sigma_e	5.4933769	
rho	.70272983	(fraction of variance due to u_i)

F test that all u_i = 0: F(3061, 1263) = 2.96   Prob > F = 0.0000

In the GLS model, the error components specification means that the overall variance of the error term can be decomposed into two components, σ^2_α associated with the individual effect and σ^2_ε associated with the idiosyncratic error term. Table 11.1 gives estimates of σ_α (*sigma_u*) and σ_ε (*sigma_e*) and also reports the value of r, the intra-group correlation coefficient, which has a value of 0.585. This shows the fraction of the overall variance of the error term that can be attributed to the individual effect. The coefficients of the regression function can be interpreted in the usual way. They show, for example, that individuals with more years of schooling smoke fewer cigarettes and those with fewer years of formal schooling smoke more.

As there are only two waves, the HALS data are not well suited to the fixed effects estimator, particularly as the two waves are seven years apart. In applying the within-groups (i.e. fixed effects) estimator, any time-invariant variables, such as the individual's gender or ethnic group, are eliminated from the regression. The remaining variables are measured as deviations from the within-individual mean. Table 11.2 is included only for comparison with the random effects estimates. The fact that HALS has only two waves means that the within-groups estimator performs very poorly. The method would come into its own with a longer panel, providing more information on each individual's behaviour as it evolves over time.

Binary choices

The discussion so far has concentrated on a simple linear panel data regression model in which the dependent variable can take a continuous range of values. In practice, analysts using health surveys are more likely to be confronted with qualitative or categorical dependent variables. These make estimation of panel data models more complex. The linear specification is attractive because taking differences or mean deviations allows the individual effect to be swept from the equation. But this is no longer possible for a non-linear regression model as typically used for qualitative and categorical variables. To illustrate, consider a binary choice model:

$$E(y|x_{it}\beta, \alpha_i) = P(y_i = 1|x_{it}\beta, \alpha_i) = F(x_{it}\beta + \alpha_i). \tag{12}$$

Taking differences or mean deviations of the non-linear function F(.) will not eliminate the individual effect. This is a problem if the individual effects are expected to be correlated with the explanatory variables.

If an analyst is willing to assume that the effects and the explanatory variables are uncorrelated, then the clustering of the dependent variable can be dealt with using a random effects specification. For example, the **random effects probit** model assumes that both components of the error term are normally distributed and that both are independent of x_{it}. By assuming a specific distribution for the individual effect it is possible to write down a sample log likelihood function that allows for the correlation in the error term within individuals. This expression can be estimated using standard software, such as Stata.

Let us return to the example of the binary measure of self-assessed health, where y equals 1 if an individual reports 'excellent' or 'good' health and

Table 11.3: Pooled probit model for sah

Probit estimates				Number of obs = 14209		
				LR chi2(27) = 702.71		
				Prob > chi2 = 0.0000		
Log likelihood = −7989.9167				Pseudo R2 = 0.0421		

yvar	Coef.	Std. Err.	z	P > |z|	[95% Conf. Interval]	
male	−.0068974	.0273188	−0.25	0.801	−.0604412	.0466464
age	−.0064117	.0017746	−3.61	0.000	−.0098898	−.0029336
age2	−.0332207	.0071209	−4.67	0.000	−.0471774	−.0192641
age3	.1101963	.0215749	5.11	0.000	.0679102	.1524823
ethbawi	−.2863132	.1133627	−2.53	0.012	−.5085	−.0641265
ethipb	−.3594183	.0983905	−3.65	0.000	−.5522602	−.1665764
ethothnw	−.3499534	.1367414	−2.56	0.010	−.6179616	−.0819452
part	.1555199	.0413251	3.76	0.000	.0745242	.2365156
unemp	−.138589	.0571241	−2.43	0.015	−.2505502	−.0266278
retd	−.0461887	.0497158	−0.93	0.353	−.1436298	.0512524
stdnt	.1145091	.1323305	0.87	0.387	−.1448538	.373872
keephse	−.1218374	.0420513	−2.90	0.004	−.2042565	−.0394184
lsch14u	−.3097408	.0689802	−4.49	0.000	−.4449396	−.1745421
lsch14	−.2626227	.0416924	−6.30	0.000	−.3443383	−.180907
lsch15	−.1576634	.0342902	−4.60	0.000	−.224871	−.0904559
lsch17	.0802489	.0481798	1.67	0.096	−.0141818	.1746796
lsch18	.1988208	.0512741	3.88	0.000	.0983254	.2993162
lsch19	−.0052156	.1063857	−0.05	0.961	−.2137278	.2032966
regsc1s	.3506734	.0604204	5.80	0.000	.2322516	.4690951
regsc2	.2177603	.0333292	6.53	0.000	.1524362	.2830843
regsc3n	.0920397	.0376473	2.44	0.014	.0182524	.165827
regsc4	−.0802458	.0333909	−2.40	0.016	−.1456907	−.0148009
regsc5n	−.2028511	.0484185	−4.19	0.000	−.2977497	−.1079526
widow	−.1249198	.0439715	−2.84	0.004	−.2111024	−.0387373
single	−.1134637	.0408279	−2.78	0.005	−.1934849	−.0334425
seprd	−.2058863	.0787671	−2.61	0.009	−.3602671	−.0515056
divorce	−.1783488	.0549352	−3.25	0.001	−.2860199	−.0706777
_cons	.8050736	.0410885	19.59	0.000	.7245416	.8856057

Table 11.4: Random effects probit model for sah

Random–effects probit
Group variable (i) : serno
Random effects u_i ~ Gaussian

Log likelihood = –7734.4866

Number of obs = 14209
Number of groups = 8952
Obs per group: min = 1
avg = 1.6
max = 2
Wald chi2(27) = 468.39
Prob > chi2 = 0.0000

yvar	Coef.	Std. Err.	z	P > |z|	[95% Conf. Interval]	
male	–.0137224	.0429172	–0.32	0.749	–.0978385	.0703937
age	–.0069471	.002674	–2.60	0.009	–.012188	–.0017062
age2	–.0559292	.0105351	–5.31	0.000	–.0765777	–.0352807
age3	.1467533	.0317494	4.62	0.000	.0845256	.208981
ethbawi	–.4072376	.179303	–2.27	0.023	–.758665	–.0558103
ethipb	–.5340048	.1548172	–3.45	0.001	–.8374409	–.2305687
ethothnw	–.5189814	.218082	–2.38	0.017	–.9464143	–.0915485
part	.1804717	.0597389	3.02	0.003	.0633855	.2975578
unemp	–.1318259	.0820375	–1.61	0.108	–.2926165	.0289646
retd	–.0619076	.070894	–0.87	0.383	–.2008572	.077042
stdnt	.1960319	.189486	1.03	0.301	–.1753538	.5674175
keephse	–.1359808	.061703	–2.20	0.028	–.2569165	–.0150451
lsch14u	–.4855768	.1103036	–4.40	0.000	–.701768	–.2693857
lsch14	–.4201722	.067375	–6.24	0.000	–.5522247	–.2881197
lsch15	–.2370722	.0552643	–4.29	0.000	–.3453882	–.1287562
lsch17	.1265407	.0771395	1.64	0.101	–.02465	.2777315
lsch18	.3343847	.0825078	4.05	0.000	.1726724	.4960971
lsch19	.007423	.1705596	0.04	0.965	–.3268677	.3417137
regsc1s	.444602	.091641	4.85	0.000	.2649889	.6242151
regsc2	.2700588	.0511486	5.28	0.000	.1698094	.3703082
regsc3n	.0773983	.0570371	1.36	0.175	–.0343925	.1891891
regsc4	–.1157136	.0502118	–2.30	0.021	–.214127	–.0173003
regsc5n	–.2983758	.0728549	–4.10	0.000	–.4411687	–.1555829
widow	–.1646477	.066808	–2.46	0.014	–.2955891	–.0337064
single	–.1199239	.0627868	–1.91	0.056	–.2429838	.0031359
seprd	–.2844771	.1121935	–2.54	0.011	–.5043724	–.0645818
divorce	–.2407617	.0822965	–2.93	0.003	–.4020599	–.0794635
_cons	1.207721	.0687456	17.57	0.000	1.072982	1.34246
/lnsig2u	.1289803	.0800067		–.02783	.2857907	
sigma_u	1.066615	.0426682		.9861814	1.153609	
rho	.5322005	.0199187		.493043	.5709653	

Likelihood ratio test of rho = 0: chibar2(01) = 510.86 Prob >= chibar2 = 0.000

equals 0 if an individual reports 'fair' or 'poor' health. Now we can make use of the longitudinal element of HALS and use information from both waves of the survey. The first set of estimates, presented in Table 11.3, is for a **pooled probit** specification. This simply takes the standard probit estimator and ignores the fact that we are dealing with repeated observations. It pools all of the observations together, not allowing for the fact that individuals are measured twice. This means that the model is estimated on the basis of a wrongly specified likelihood function. However, it can be shown that the estimator does give consistent estimates of the population-averaged coefficients, even though it ignores the structure of the error term. However, robust standard errors should be used that allow for the clustering of observations within individuals. Compare these estimates with the cross-section results for the **probit model** in Chapter 3. Now we have a larger sample because we are using information from wave 2 as well as wave 1. Again, the coefficients should be interpreted as qualitative effects and quantitative inferences should be made on the basis of average or marginal effects. Once more, we can see clear gradients in self-assessed health by education and by occupational socioeconomic group.

Table 11.4 shows the **random effects probit** model. The table includes an estimate of ρ, the intra-group correlation coefficient. This suggests that the individual effect accounts for around half (0.532) of the random variation.

Recall that the random effects probit model embodies two important assumptions: that the individual effect has a normal distribution and that it is uncorrelated with the explanatory variables. The first assumption can be relaxed by using a **semiparametric** approach. For example Deb (2001) develops a **finite mixture random effects probit** model, using the same sort of methods that were described in Chapters 9 and 10.

The second assumption – that the individual effects are uncorrelated with the explanatory variables – can be dealt with in two ways. The first is to adopt a **fixed effects** specification, treating the individual effects as parameters to be estimated, or at least eliminated from the model. The second is to use a **correlated random effects** specification. It has already been stressed that, for most non-linear models, the convenient device for taking mean deviations or first differences is no longer feasible. This is certainly the case for the panel data probit model. However, the **logit** model is an exception to this rule. Because of the special features of the logistic function, it is possible to reformulate the model in a way that eliminates the individual effect, α. This is known as the **conditional logit** model. For example when there are only two waves in the panel ($T = 2$), by restricting attention to those individuals who change status during the course of the panel, it is possible to estimate the standard logit model using first differences in the explanatory variables, rather than the levels of the variables. This means that the standard logit model can be applied to differenced data and the individual effect is swept out in the process. Like the fixed effects estimator for linear models, this approach will work well only if there is sufficient within-individual variation in the variables.

Another approach to dealing with individual random effects that are correlated with the explanatory variables is to specify this relationship directly, for example by specifying this relationship as a linear regression of the value of the explanatory variables in all of the waves of the panel. A convenient special case of this approach includes only within-individual means of the regressors. This function is then substituted back into the original equation and, as long as there is sufficient within-individual variation, it allows separate estimates of the βs and of the correlation between the x variables and the individual effect to be disentangled (*see* the Technical appendix and Jones 2000 for details of this method). In this sense, this method has a strong parallel with the within-group estimator.

Attrition bias

Using panel data – such as the Health and Lifestyle Survey (HALS) and other panels such as the British Household Panel Survey (BHPS) or European Community Household Panel (ECHP) – to analyse longitudinal models of health creates a risk that the results will be contaminated by bias associated with longitudinal non-response. There are drop-outs from the panels at each wave and some of these may be related directly to health: due to deaths, serious illness and people moving into institutional care. In addition, other sources of non-response may be indirectly related to health, for example divorce may increase the risk of non-response and also be associated with poorer health than average. The long-term survivors who remain in the panel are likely to be healthier on average compared to the sample at wave 1. The health of survivors will tend to be higher than the population as a whole and their rate of decline in health will tend to be lower. Also, the socioeconomic status of the survivors may not be representative of the original population who were sampled at wave 1.

A broad definition of longitudinal non-response encompasses any observations that 'drop out' from the original sample over the subsequent T waves. Non-response can arise due to:

1 demographic events such as death
2 movement out of the scope of the survey, such as institutionalisation or emigration
3 refusal to respond at subsequent waves
4 absence of the person at the address
5 other types of non-contact.

The notion of attrition, commonly used in the survey methods literature, is often restricted to points 3, 4 and 5. However, our concern is with any longitudinal non-response that leads to missing observations in the panel data regression analysis. In fact it is points 1 and 2 – death and incapacity – that are likely to be most relevant as sources of health-related non-response.

Testing

A simple variable addition test can be used to diagnose attrition bias in panel data regressions. This involves adding a test variable that reflects non-response, to the original regression model and testing its significance. The test variables that can be used are: (i) an indicator for whether the individual responds in the subsequent wave; (ii) an indicator of whether the individual responds in all waves and, hence, is in the balanced sample; and (iii) a count of the number of waves that are observed for the individual. The t-ratios on the added variables provide three variants of the test for non-response bias. The intuition behind these tests is that, if non-response is random, indicators of an individual's pattern of survey responses should not be associated with the outcome of interest after controlling for the observed covariates. Additional evidence can be provided by Hausman-type tests that compare estimates from the balanced sample, for whom we have complete information at all waves, and the unbalanced sample, for whom we have incomplete information for some individuals. In the absence of non-response bias these estimates should be comparable, but non-response bias may affect the unbalanced and balanced samples differently, leading to a contrast between the estimates. It should be noted that the variable addition tests and Hausman-type tests may have low power to detect the problem of attrition bias as they rely on the sample of observed outcomes and will not capture non-response associated with idiosyncratic shocks that are not reflected in observed outcomes.

Estimation

One approach to dealing with attrition bias is to adopt the selection on unobservables framework and use variants of the sample selection model described in Chapter 7. Here we concentrate on an alternative approach, based on selection on observables. To allow for non-response we can adopt an **inverse probability weighted (IPW)** estimator. This approach is grounded in the notion of missing at random, or ignorable, non-response. Using R as an indicator of response (R = 1 if observed, 0 otherwise) and y and x as the outcome and covariates of interest: missing completely at random (MCAR) is defined by $P(R = 1|y,x) = P(R = 1)$ and missing at random (MAR) is defined by $P(R = 1|y,x) = P(R = 1|x)$. The latter implies that, after conditioning on observed covariates, the probability of non-response does not vary systematically with the outcome of interest.

Fitzgerald *et al.* (1998) extend the notion of ignorable non-response by introducing the concepts of selection on observables and selection on unobservables. This requires an additional set of observables, z, that are available in the data but not included in the regression model. Selection on observables is defined by Fitzgerald *et al.* by the conditional independence condition $P(R = 1|y, x, z) = P(R = 1|x,z)$. Selection on unobservables occurs if this conditional independence assumption does not hold. Selection on unobservables, also termed informative, non-random or non-ignorable non-response, is familiar in the econometrics literature where the dominant approach to non-response follows the sample selection model. This approach relies on the z being 'instruments' that are good predictors of non-response and that satisfy the exclusion restriction $P(y|x,z) = P(y|x)$. This is quite different from the selection on observables approach that seeks z-values which are endogenous to y. Also it is worth mentioning that linear fixed effects panel estimators are consistent, in the presence of selection on unobservables, so long as the non-ignorable non-response is due to time invariant unobservables.

The validity of the selection on observables approach hinges on whether the conditional independence assumption holds and non-response can be treated as ignorable, once z is controlled for. If the condition does hold, consistent estimates can be obtained by weighting the observed data by the inverse of the probability of response, conditional on the observed covariates. This gives more weight to individuals who have a high probability of non-response, as they are under-represented in the observed sample. Fitzgerald *et al.* (1998) make it clear that this approach will be applicable when interest centres on a structural model for P(y|x) and that the z-values are deliberately excluded from the model, even though they are endogenous to the outcome of interest. They suggest lagged dependent variables as an obvious candidate for z. Of course, this approach will breakdown if an individual suffers an unobserved health shock, that occurs after their previous interview, that leads them to drop out of the survey and that is not captured by conditioning on lagged measures. In this case non-response would remain non-ignorable even after conditioning on z.

It is possible to test the validity of the selection on observables approach. The first step is to test whether the z-values do predict non-response; this is done by testing their significance in the **probit** models for non-response at each wave of the panel. The second is to do **Hausman**-type tests to compare the coefficients from the weighted and unweighted estimates. Finally an inversion test can be used: conditioning on patterns of response by splitting the sample into those in the balanced panel and the drop-outs and then comparing models for the dependent variable in the initial wave estimated on the subsamples.

Appendix: Stata code for panel data models

To analyse panel data, Stata needs to be given the individual identifier (i) and the time identifier (t) and the data has to be sorted by these variables. In the HALS these are given by the variables 'serno' and 'wave':

```
iis serno
tis wave
sort serno wave
```

It is useful to create indicators of whether observations are in the balanced and in the unbalanced estimation samples and a variable that records the number of waves for each observation (T_i). This is done by running a regression model for fagday and exploiting 'e(sample)', an indicator of whether or not an observation was used in the estimation of the previous model that is saved automatically by Stata:

```
Replace yvar=fagday
quietly regr yvar $xvars, robust cluster(pid)
gen insampm = 0
recode insampm 0 = 1 if e(sample)
sort serno wave
gen constant = 1
by serno: egen Ti = sum(constant) if insampm == 1
drop constant
sort wave
by serno: gen nextwavem = insampm[_n+1]
gen allwavesm = .
recode allwavesm . = 0 if Ti ~= 2
recode allwavesm . = 1 if Ti == 2
gen numwavesm = .
replace numwavesm = Ti
```

To estimate correlated effects specifications of the regressions of the regression models we need the within-individual means of the x variables. This is illustrated here for 'unemp':

```
by serno: egen munemp=mean(unemp)
```

The full set of these variables is added to the variable list to create a new global $xvarsm (not shown here).

Linear models for panel data

We begin by estimating linear panel data specifications for the number of cigarettes smoked per day ('fagday'). Before estimating any regression models it is helpful to summarise the data using 'xtsum', a command that takes account of the panel structure and analyses the variables according to their between and within variation:

```
xtsum yvar $xvars
```

The first regression model is a simple pooled OLS regression that effectively treats the panel as one big cross-section dataset and does not take account of the clustering of observations within individuals:

```
regr yvar $xvars
```

This can be augmented with robust standard errors that allow for the clustering:

```
regr yvar $xvars, robust cluster(serno)
```

Both models are re-estimated using $xvarsm, that adds within-individual means of the time-varying regressors to allow for correlated individual effects:

```
regr yvar $xvarsm
regr yvar $xvarsm, robust cluster(serno)
```

The panel data structure of the data is modelled explicitly in the **random effects (RE)** model, which assumes that there is a time invariant individual random effect. For consistency it must be assumed that this effect is independent of the regressors. The model is complemented by a **Lagrange multiplier (LM) test** of the joint significance of the individual effects and a **Hausman test** that compares the random effects with the **fixed effects** estimates. The latter provides a test of the assumption that the individual effects are uncorrelated with the regressors:

```
xtreg yvar $xvars, re
* LM TEST FOR SIGNIFICANCE OF INDIVIDUAL EFFECTS
xttest0
* HAUSMAN TEST FOR RE V. FE COEFFICIENTS
xthaus
```

All of the models above have been estimated on all available observations, that is on the unbalanced panel. Now they are re-estimated on the balanced panel, those observations who appear at every wave:

```
xtreg yvar $xvars if allwavesm==1, re
xttest0
xthaus
```

The random effects model can be augmented with $xvarsm as well. This is an alternative to the fixed effects model as a way of relaxing the assumption of uncorrelated effects. The Hausman tests from this specification can be compared to the ones carried out earlier:

```
xtreg yvar $xvarsm, re
xthaus
xtreg yvar $xvarsm if allwavesm==1, re
xthaus
```

Moving on now to the **fixed effects (FE)** specification. The direct way of estimating this model is to include a dummy variable for each individual – the least squares dummy variable (LSDV) estimator. This is automated in Stata by the 'areg' command:

```
areg yvar $xvars, absorb(serno)
```

Once the model has been run, predictions of the individual effect can be obtained and regressed on time invariant regressors, '$zvars', to explore the association between the individual effect and observable characteristics:

```
predict ai, d
regress ai $zvars if wave==1
```

The more usual way of estimating the fixed effects model is to use the within estimator, based on mean deviations. Here this is done for both the unbalanced and balanced panels:

```
xtreg yvar $xvars, fe
xtreg yvar $xvars if allwavesm==1, fe
```

To complete the trinity of panel data estimators (random, fixed and between) we estimate the **between effects (BE) model**. This model is rarely used in practice:

```
xtreg yvar $xvars, be
```

Nonlinear models for panel data

To illustrate nonlinear models for panel data we move to the binary measure of self-assessed health, 'sah':

```
replace yvar=sah
xtsum yvar $xvars
xtsum yvar $xvars if allwavesm==1
```

The first model to estimate is the pooled **probit** model, using robust standard errors to exploit the **pseudo-maximum likelihood** property of this estimator. 'dprobit' is used to compute the **partial effects** directly. Individual-specific partial effects could be computed by adapting the code presented for cross-section probit models above. Estimates are computed for the unbalanced and balanced samples and with and without $xvarsm:

```
dprobit yvar $xvars, robust cluster(serno)
dprobit yvar $xvars if allwavesm==1, robust cluster(serno)
dprobit yvar $xvarsm, robust cluster(serno)
dprobit yvar $xvarsm if allwavesm==1, robust cluster(serno)
```

While the pooled model uses the cross-section probit command, the **random effects probit** model uses the specialised command 'xtprobit'. The model is estimated by quadrature to deal with the numerical integration involved. It is wise to use the 'quadchk' command to verify that sufficient evaluation points have been used in the quadrature routine. If not, the number of points can be increased. Estimates are computed for the unbalanced and balanced samples and with and without the $xvarsm:

```
xtprobit yvar $xvars
quadchk
xtprobit yvar $xvars if allwavesm==1
quadchk
xtprobit yvar $xvarsm
quadchk
xtprobit yvar $xvarsm if allwavesm==1
quadchk
```

Finally, we estimate the **conditional logit** model:

```
clogit yvar $xvars, group(serno)
clogit yvar $xvars if allwavesm==1, group(serno)
```

Concluding thoughts

This book has illustrated the diversity of applied econometric methods that are available to health economists who work with microdata. The text has emphasised the range of models and estimators that are available, but that should not imply a neglect of the need for sound economic theory and careful data collection to produce worthwhile econometric research. Most of the methods reviewed here are designed for individual-level data. Because of the widespread use of observational data in health economics, particular care should be devoted to dealing with problems of self-selection and unobservable heterogeneity. This is likely to set the agenda for future research, with the emphasis on robust estimators applied to panel data and other complex data sets.

Further reading

General

Cameron AC, Trivedi PK. *Microeconometrics. Methods and applications*. Cambridge University Press; 2005.

Deaton A. *The Analysis of Household Surveys: a microeconometric approach to development policy*. Johns Hopkins University Press for the World Bank; 1997.

Greene WH. *Econometric Analysis*. 4th ed. Prentice Hall; 2000.

Jones AM. Health econometrics. In: Culyer AJ, Newhouse JP, editors. *Handbook of Health Economics*. Elsevier; 2000.

Jones AM, O'Donnell OA. *Econometric Analysis of Health Data*. Wiley; 2001.

Verbeek M. *Modern Econometrics*. 2nd ed. Wiley; 2004.

Wooldridge J. *Econometric Analysis of Cross Section and Panel Data*. The MIT Press; 2002.

Qualitative dependent variables

Gourieroux C. *Econometrics of Qualitative Dependent Variables*. Cambridge University Press; 2000.

Maddala GS. *Limited Dependent and Qualitative Variables in Econometrics*. Cambridge University Press; 1983.

Pudney S. *Modelling Individual Choice: the econometrics of corners, kinks and holes*. Blackwell; 1989.

Train KE. *Discrete Choice Methods with Simulation*. Cambridge University Press; 2003.

Sample selection and the evaluation problem

Auld MC. Using observational data to identify causal effects of health-related behaviour. In: Jones AM, editor. *Elgar Companion to Health Economics*. Edward Elgar; 2006.

Polsky D, Basu A. Selection bias in observational data. In: Jones AM, editor. *Elgar Companion to Health Economics*. Edward Elgar; 2006.

Vella F. Estimating models with sample selection bias. *J Human Res*. 1998; **33**: 127–69.

Count data

Cameron AC, Trivedi PK. *Regression Analysis of Count Data*. Cambridge University Press; 1998.

Deb P, Trivedi PK. Empirical models of health care use. In: Jones AM, editor. *Elgar Companion to Health Economics*. Edward Elgar; 2006.

Duration analysis

Lancaster T. *The Econometric Analysis of Transition Data*. Cambridge University Press; 1992.

Panel data (and multilevel models)

Arellano M. *Panel Data Econometrics*. Oxford University Press; 2003.

Baltagi BH. *Econometric Analysis of Panel Data*. 3rd ed. Wiley; 2005.

Contoyannis P, Jones AM, Leon-Gonzalez R. Using simulation-based inference with panel data in health economics. *Health Econ*. 2004; **13**: 101–22.

Rice N, Jones AM. Multilevel models and health economics. *Health Econ*. 1997; **6**(6): 561–75.

Glossary

Asymptotic property

A property of a statistic that applies as the sample size grows large (specifically, as it tends to infinity).

Attrition bias

Bias caused by unit non-response in panel data. This occurs when the individuals who drop out of a panel study are systematically different from those who remain in it.

Average effect

A measure of the effect of a binary explanatory variable, x, on the outcome of interest; based on comparing the outcome when x equals 1 with the outcome when x equals 0.

Average treatment effect (ATE)

A measure commonly used in the policy evaluation literature that gives the expected difference in outcomes between those who receive a treatment and those who do not, across the whole study population. Related to the average treatment effect on the treated (ATET), which is the expected difference for those who would opt for treatment.

Between effects (BE) model

An approach to panel data estimation that only uses the (cross-section) variation between individuals, not variation within individuals.

Binary variable

A variable that takes only two values, usually coded as zero and one.

Bivariate probit

A model that combines two binary probit models to deal with a system of two binary dependent variables.

Conditional logit

A model for unordered multinomial outcomes in which the regressors vary across the alternatives (*see* mixed logit and multinomial logit).

Consistent estimate

An estimate that converges on the true parameter value as the sample size increases (towards infinity).

Continuous variable

A variable that can take the value of any real number within an interval.

Correlated random effects

A variant of the random effects (RE) approach to panel data that allows the individual effect to be correlated with the observed regressors.

Cox proportional hazard model

A semiparametric model for duration analysis.

Cross-section survey data

Survey data in which each respondent is observed only once, giving a 'snapshot' view of the population at a point in time.

Dummy variable

Another label for binary variables that take the value zero or one.

Equi-dispersion

When the mean and variance are equal. Arises in the context of count data regression. *See* over-dispersion and under-dispersion.

Error components model

A regression model for panel data.

Excess zeros

A feature of count data, when the number of zeroes observed exceeds the number that would be expected from the Poisson model.

Exogeneity

In the context of regression analysis, the assumption that the regressors, x, are independent of the error term.

Finite mixture model

A mixture model (*see* below) in which the heterogeneity has a discrete distribution.

Fixed effects (FE)

The fixed effects specification treats the individual effects in panel data models as parameters to be estimated. This is appropriate when inferences are to be confined to the effects in the sample only, and the effects themselves are of substantive interest. With individual-level survey data, fixed effects are best interpreted as random individual effects that are correlated with the explanatory variables. This contrasts with random effects that are assumed to be independent of the regressors (*see* random effects).

Full-information maximum likelihood (FIML)

Estimates multiple equation models using the joint distribution for the equations rather than estimating each equation separately.

Gamma distribution

Probability distribution often used to model individual heterogeneity, especially in count data regression and duration analysis.

Generalised least squares (GLS)

A generalisation of ordinary least squares which relaxes the assumption that the error terms are independently and identically distributed across observations.

Generalised method of moments (GMM)

Many of the estimators discussed in this book fall within the unifying framework of generalised method of moments (GMM) estimation. This replaces population moment conditions (e.g. based on expected values) with their sample analogues (e.g. based on sample means).

Grouped data regression   *See* interval regression.

Hausman test   Tests whether there is a significant difference between two sets of coefficients: one set that is efficient under the null but inconsistent under the alternative and another set that is inefficient under the null but still consistent under the alternative. Commonly used to test the IIA assumption in multinomial choice models and as a test of exogeneity (comparing OLS and IV estimates).

Hazard function   Defined as the ratio of the density function to the survivor function for a random variable. The hazard function plays a key role in duration analysis where it is interpreted as the probability of failing now given survival up to now.

Heckit model   A two-step estimator designed to deal with the sample selection problem.

Heteroskedasticity   When the variance of the error term is not constant across observations.

Homoskedasticity   When the variance of the error term is constant across observations.

Hurdle models   Models, often used with count data, that split the dependent variable into two parts: a probability of participating and the number of events, such as doctor visits, conditional on participating.

Instrumental variables (IV)   A method of estimation for models with endogenous regressors – regressors that are correlated with the error term. It relies on variables (or 'instruments') that are good predictors of an endogenous regressor, but are not independently related to the dependent variable. These may be used to purge the bias caused by endogeneity.

Interval regression   A variant on the ordered probit model that can be used when the threshold values are known. *See also* grouped data regression.

Inverse Mills ratio (IMR)   The label given to the hazard rate (ratio of density to survival functions) for a probit model. The IMR is used in the Heckit correction for sample selection bias.

Inverse probability weights (IPW)	Used to reweight sample data to make them representative of the underlying population. IPWs give more weight to those observations that are under-represented in the sample.
Item non-response	When a respondent does not provide data for a particular variable in a survey.
Kaplan-Meier	A nonparametric estimator for survival curves and hazard functions.
Lagrange multiplier (LM) test	A method of testing hypotheses, expressed as restrictions on parameters, that only requires estimates under the null model, with the restrictions imposed. This can be convenient if the unrestricted model is hard to estimate.
Left truncation	A phenomenon that arises with duration data that have been sampled after the original start of the process. Left truncation occurs when some observations may have already failed before the data are collected and are therefore missing from the data.
Likelihood ratio (LR) tests	LR statistics are used to test hypotheses, in the form of restrictions on parameters, with maximum likelihood estimators. The LR statistic compares the value of the log-likelihood when estimation is uncon-strained to the value when the parameters are restricted. Twice the difference between the log-likelihood values has a chi-squared distribution, which can be used to assess the statistical significance of the test statistic. The degrees of freedom for the statistic are given by the number of restrictions to be tested.
Linear probability model	A model for binary dependent variables based on the linear regression model.
Logistic distribution	A continuous probability distribution that is the foundation for the logit model of binary choice.
Logit	A model for binary dependent variables based on the logistic distribution.
Marginal effect	A measure of the effect of a continuous explanatory variable, x, on the outcome of interest; based on the derivative of the outcome with respect to x.
Maximum likelihood (ML) estimation	A method of estimation that specifies the joint probability of the observed set of data and finds the parameter values that maximise it (i.e. that are most likely).

Mixed logit	A model for unordered multinomial outcomes in which the regressors can vary across individuals and across the choices. The label is also applied to the more general random parameters logit model. (*See* conditional logit and multinomial logit).
Mixture models	A general class of models that combine two separate probabilty distributions. Often used to incorporate individual heterogeneity, for example when a gamma distribution for heterogeneity is mixed with the Poisson distribution to produce the negbin model.
Multinomial logit	A model for unordered multinomial outcomes in which the regressors vary across individuals (*see* mixed logit and conditional logit).
Negbin	Negative binomial – an extension of the Poisson regression model for count data.
Nelson-Aalen	A nonparametric estimator for cumulative hazard functions.
Normal distribution	A continuous probabilty distribution that has a typical 'bell shape'. Used as the foundation for classical regression and analysis and many other models such as the probit model and the Heckit model.
Ordered probit	A model for ordered multinomial outcomes.
Ordinary least squares (OLS)	The standard method for fitting the classical linear regression model. It is based on finding the parameter values that minimise the sum of squared errors.
Over-dispersion	When observed count data are more spread out than would be expected from a Poisson model.
Panel data	Survey data in which each respondent is observed repeatedly over time.
Partial effect	Used to measure the impact of a change in a regressor on the probability of the outcome of interest. Relevant for non-linear models, such as binary choice models, where the partial effect is not simply the regression coefficient.
Point estimate	A single number used to estimate an unknown parameter (the 'best guess'). As opposed to an interval estimate, which presents a range of values.
Poisson regression	A model for count data.

Pooled probit	When a standard probit model is applied to panel data.
Probit	A model for binary dependent variables based on the standard normal distribution.
Propensity score	The probability of participating (in a treatment) conditional on a set of regressors, $p(y = 1|x)$. The propensity score is used in matching and sample selection estimators.
Pseudo maximum likelihood estimation	A property of certain models, that maximum likelihood estimates are still consistent even when the likelihood function is misspecified. For example, the Poisson regression estimator has this property so long as the mean of the distribution is correctly specified even if the variance is not.
Pseudo R-squareds	A label for measures of goodness of fit used for nonlinear regression models, such as binary choice and count data models. Called pseudo because, unlike the linear regression model, the identity that total variation equals explained plus unexplained variation does not hold.
Qualitative effect	The sign of the effect of one variable on another.
Quantitative effect	The magnitude of the effect of one variable on another.
Random effects (RE)	The random effects specification treats the individual effects in panel data models as random draws. If individual effects are not of intrinsic importance in themselves and are assumed to be random draws from a population of individuals, and if inferences concerning population effects and their characteristics are sought, then a random specification is suitable (*see* fixed effects).
Random effects probit	A model for binary dependent variables in panel data.
RESET	A general test for misspecification of the functional form of a regression model.
Retransformation problem	Highlights the need to use an appropriate transformation back to the y-scale when regression models are run on transformed data such as $\log(y)$.
Right censoring	Occurs when values in the right-hand tail of a distribution are cut off at some threshold and only the threshold value is

	known. This often arises in duration analysis where some spells are incomplete at the time the data are collected.
Robust estimator	An estimator that is robust to general assumptions and model misspecification. For example robust estimates of standard errors allow for heteroskedasticity while standard estimates do not.
Sample selection bias	The bias created when non-responders are systematically different from responders.
Semiparametric	A method that mixes parametric assumptions (e.g. that the relationship between y and x is linear) and non-parametric assumptions (e.g. that the distribution of the error term is unknown).
Serial independence	Relates to the properties of time series variables, such as error terms from regression models, and means that current values are independent of past and future values.
Split population model	A specification used with duration data that splits the population into potential and non-potential participants.
Under-dispersion	When observed count data are less spread out than would be expected from a Poisson model.
Unit non-response	When a potential respondent does not provide data for any variables in a survey.
Unbalanced panel	A panel dataset that includes all respondents who report data for at least one period (wave) of the panel. In contrast to a balanced panel which only includes those individuals with complete data for all periods.
Weibull model	A parametric model for duration analysis.
Weighted least squares(WLS)	Weights (w_i) are attached to the values of the dependent variable (y_i) and independent variable (x_i) before using least squares regression. This method can be used to correct for heteroskedasticity.
Zero-inflated models	A version of count data regression that adds extra weight to the probability of a zero observation.

Technical appendix

Maximum likelihood estimation (MLE)

A simple example

To give an example of MLE, consider an i.i.d. sample of Bernoulli trials, where each of the trials has an outcome of 0 or 1:

$$y_i = 1 \text{ with probability } \beta, \text{ and } = 0 \text{ with probability } 1 - \beta.$$

Given a sample of n observations: with n_0 zeros and n_1 ones. These have joint probability:

$$P(y_{1 \ldots} y_n \mid \beta) = (1 - \beta) \ldots (1 - \beta) \beta \ldots \beta = (1 - \beta)^{n_0}\beta^{n_1}.$$

Reinterpret this as a sample likelihood function:

$$L(\beta|y) = (1 - \beta)^{n_0}\beta^{n_1},$$

with sample log-likelihood function:

$$l(\beta|y) = \log\{L(\beta|y)\} = n_0\log(1 - \beta) + n_1\log(\beta).$$

Then find the MLE of β as the value that maximises $l(\beta|y)$. The first order condition is:

$$d(\beta) = \partial l(\beta|y)/\partial\beta = -n_0/(1 - \beta) + n_1/(\beta) = 0,$$

where $\partial l(\beta|y)/\partial\beta$ is known as the score function. This solves to give:

$$\beta_{mle} = n_1/n.$$

So, in this case, the MLE is the sample proportion.

Some general theory for MLE

Discrete y:

$$L(\beta|y) = \Pi \, P(y| \, \beta)$$

$$l(\beta|y) = \Sigma \, \text{Log}P(y| \, \beta).$$

Continuous y:

$$L(\beta|y) = \Pi \, f(y|\beta)$$

$$l(\beta|y) = \Sigma \, \log f(y|\beta).$$

The maximum likelihood estimator is:

$$\beta_{mle} = b = \text{argmax } l(\beta|y).$$

The estimator is consistent and asymptotically normal.

Binary responses

When y equals 0 or 1, the conditional expectation of y is:

$$E(y_i|x_i) = P(y_i = 1|x_i) = F(x_i).$$

The most common nonlinear parametric specifications are logit and probit models. These can be given a latent variable interpretation. Let:

$$y_i = 1 \text{ if } y^*_i > 0$$

$$= 0 \text{ otherwise}$$

where,

$$y^*_i = x_i\beta + \varepsilon_i.$$

Then:

$$P(y_i = 1| x_i) = P(y^*_i > 0|x_i) = P(\varepsilon_i > -x_i\beta) = F(x_i\beta).$$

The log-likelihood for a sample of independent observations is:

$$\text{LogL} = \Sigma_i \{(1 - y_i)\log(1 - F(x_i\beta)) + y_i \log(F(x_i\beta))\}.$$

Multinomial and ordered responses

Ordered probit

The ordered probit model can be used to model a discrete dependent variable that takes ordered multinomial outcomes, e.g. y = 1, 2 ... , m.

$$y_i = j \text{ if } \mu_{j-1} < y^*_i \le \mu_j, j = 1, ..., m$$

where,

$$y^*_i = x_i\beta + \varepsilon_i, \varepsilon_i \sim N(0,1)$$

and $\mu_0 = -\infty, \mu_j \le \mu_{j+1}, \mu_m = \infty$.

$$P_{ij} = P(y_i = j) = \Phi(\mu_j - x_i\beta) - \Phi(\mu_{j-1} - x_i\beta).$$

The log-likelihood takes the form,

$$\text{LogL} = \Sigma_i \Sigma_j y_{ij} \log P_{ij}$$

where y_{ij} is a binary variable that equals 1 if $y_i = j$.

Multinomial logit

Multinomial models apply to discrete dependent variables that can take (unordered) multinomial outcomes, $y = 1, 2, \dots, m$. Define a set of binary variables to indicate which alternative ($j = 1, \dots, m$) is chosen by each individual ($I = 1, \dots, n$),

$$y_{ij} = 1 \text{ if } y_i = j$$

$$= 0 \text{ otherwise}$$

with associated probabilities,

$$P(y_i = j) = P_{ij}.$$

With independent observations, the log-likelihood for a multinomial model takes the form:

$$\text{LogL} = \Sigma_i \, \Sigma_j \, y_{ij} \log P_{ij}.$$

The multinomial logit model uses:

$$P_{ij} = \exp(x_i\beta_j) \, / \, \Sigma_k \exp(x_i\beta_k)$$

with a normalisation that $\beta_m = 0$.

Bivariate probit

The bivariate probit model applies to a pair of binary dependent variables:

$$y^*_{ji} = x_{ji}\beta_j + \varepsilon_j, \, j = 1, 2, \, (\varepsilon_1, \varepsilon_2) \sim N(0, \Omega)$$

where,

$$y_{ji} = 1 \text{ if } y^*_{ji} > 0$$

$$= 0 \text{ otherwise.}$$

The sample selection model

It is possible to express the sample selection model in terms of latent variables (y^*):

$$y^*_{ji} = x_{ji}\beta_j + \varepsilon_j, \, j = 1, 2.$$

Then the sample selection model is given by:

$$y_i = y^*_{2i} \text{ if } y^*_{1i} > 0$$

$$= \text{unobserved otherwise.}$$

Endogenous regressors and the evaluation problem

Selection on observables: the recursive bivariate probit model

The bivariate probit model applies to a pair of binary dependent variables and allows for correlation between the corresponding error terms. In our application, the use of visits to a medical specialist is modelled as a recursive bivariate probit model. The model consists of two latent variable equations for insurance and specialist visits:

$$y_{1i}^* = \alpha' x_i + \eta' w_i + \varepsilon_{1i}$$

$$y_{2i}^* = \gamma y_{1i} + \beta' x_i + \varepsilon_{2i}$$

where

$$(\varepsilon_1, \varepsilon_2) \sim N(0, \Omega)$$

and

$$y_j = 1 \text{ if } y^*_j > 0$$

$$= 0 \text{ otherwise}$$

The identification strategy relies on the fact that we are modelling sequential decisions. Estimation of the model by FIML, taking account of the joint distribution of ε_1 and ε_2 deals with the endogeneity of y_1. The log-likelihood for the model is:

$$\log L = \sum_{i=1}^{n} \log\{\Phi\{(\alpha' x_i + \eta' w_i), d_2(\gamma y_{1i} + \beta' x_i), d_{1i} d_{2i}\rho\}\}$$

where $\Phi[.]$ is the bivariate normal CDF, $d_j = 2y_j - 1$ and ρ is the coefficient of correlation between ε_1 and ε_2. The asymptotic t-ratio for the estimate of ρ provides a test for exogeneity.

A more general approach to FIML estimation

To allow for potential selection effects the treatment (y_1) and outcome (y_2) may be modelled jointly in a recursive specification. The model assumes that the treatment has a direct causal effect on the outcome and that both are influenced by common unobservable factors:

$$y_{1i} = \beta_1 x_{1i} + \varepsilon_{1i}$$

$$y_{2i} = \alpha y_{1i} + \beta_2 x_{2i} + \varepsilon_{2i}.$$

A common factor specification of the error terms can be used to allow for selection effects. So:

$$\varepsilon_{1i} = \rho_1 v_i + u_{1i}$$

$$\varepsilon_{2i} = \rho_2 v_i + u_{2i}.$$

Given this specification, unobserved heterogeneity can be dealt with by integrating v out:

$$f(\varepsilon_{1i}, \varepsilon_{2i}) = \int_{-\infty}^{\infty} f(\varepsilon_{1i}, \varepsilon_{2i}|v) dF(v),$$

where $f(\varepsilon_{1i}, \varepsilon_{2i})$ denotes the joint distribution of ε_1 and ε_{2i}, $f(\varepsilon_{1i}, \varepsilon_{2i}|v)$ denotes their joint distribution conditional on v and F(v) denotes the marginal distribution function of v. Given independence of u_1 and u_2, this simplifies to:

$$f(\varepsilon_{1i}, \varepsilon_{2i}) = \int_{-\infty}^{\infty} f(\varepsilon_{1i}|v) f(\varepsilon_{2i}|v) dF(v),$$

which can be used to form the sample likelihood function:

$$L_i = \int_{-\infty}^{\infty} \{g(v)\} dF(v) = \int_{-\infty}^{\infty} \{g(v)\} f(v) \, dv,$$

where g(.) is formed as the product of the marginal distributions and is a complex nonlinear function of v. Computation of the likelihood function requires evaluation of this integral. Possible estimators include Gauss-Hermite quadrature, maximum simulated likelihood (MSL) and the finite density estimator.

Gauss-Hermite quadrature

The conventional approach to evaluating likelihood functions is numerical integration by quadrature. Examples include the random effects probit model and count data regressions with endogenous binary regressors. To use Gauss-Hermite quadrature, assume $v \sim N(0, \sigma^2)$. Then the likelihood function takes the form:

$$L_i = \int_{-\infty}^{\infty} (1/\sqrt{2\pi\sigma^2}) \, \exp(-v^2/2\sigma^2) \, \{g(v)\} dv.$$

Use a change of variable, $v = (\sqrt{2\sigma^2})z$, to give:

$$L_i = (1/\sqrt{\pi}) \int_{-\infty}^{\infty} \exp(-z^2) \, \{g((\sqrt{2\sigma^2})z)\} dz.$$

This form of the integrand is suitable for Gauss-Hermite quadrature. Hence the integral can be approximated by the weighted sum:

$$L_i \approx (1/\sqrt{\pi}) \sum_{j=1}^{m} w_j \, g((\sqrt{2\sigma^2})a_j).$$

The weights (w_j) and ordinates (a_j) are tabulated in standard references and automated in software packages such as Stata.

Maximum simulated likelihood (MSL)

An alternative to quadrature is to approximate the likelihood using Monte Carlo integration and estimate the parameters by the method of maximum simulated likelihood (MSL). Estimation by simulation is not necessary in the case of a univariate integral, but it would come into its own with a multiple factor specification.

The aim is to simulate the sample likelihood function:

$$L_i = \int_{-\infty}^{\infty} \{g(v)\} f(v) dv.$$

Again assume $v \sim N(0, \sigma^2)$. Then:

$$L_i = \int_{-\infty}^{\infty} (1/\sqrt{2\pi\sigma^2}) \exp(-v^2/2\sigma^2) \{g(v)\} dv.$$

In this case use the change of variable, $z = v/\sigma$, to give:

$$L_i = \int_{-\infty}^{\infty} (1/\sqrt{2\pi}) \exp(-\tfrac{1}{2}z^2) \{g(\sigma z)\} dz.$$

So:

$$L_i = \int_{-\infty}^{\infty} \phi(z) \{q(z)\} dz,$$

where $\phi(z)$ denotes the standard normal pdf, and $q(z) = g(\sigma z)$. This is the expected value of $h(z)$ with respect to z:

$$= E_z [q(z)]$$

The principle behind MSL estimation is to replace this population expectation with a sample analogue. The individual contribution to the simulated likelihood function is:

$$L_i = (1/R) \sum_{j=1}^{m} q(z_j),$$

where the z-values are draws from a standard normal distribution and the simulated likelihood is the average of $q(z_j)$ over R draws. The MSL estimator is consistent as both n and R go to infinity, but is biased for fixed R.

Finite density estimators

Gauss-Hermite quadrature and MSL estimation both rely on an assumption about the parametric form of the density of v. An alternative, semiparametric, approach is provided by the finite density estimator.

The idea of the finite density estimator is to approximate the unknown density $f(v)$ in:

$$L_i = \int_{-\infty}^{\infty} \{g(v)\} f(v) dv$$

by a set of discrete mass points. This gives the quasi-likelihood function:

$$L_i = \sum_{j=1}^{k} \pi_j g(\eta_j),$$

where the π_js and η_js are estimated along with the other parameters. The number of mass points is selected using statistical criteria. Typically 2–5 points are used. The π_js must satisfy the conditions

$$0 \le \pi_j \le 1 \quad \forall j$$

and

$$\sum_{j=1}^{k} \pi_j = 1.$$

In practice, these can be imposed by using a logistic parameterisation:

$$\pi_j = \exp(\omega_j)/\Sigma \exp(\omega_k)$$

and estimating the ω_js.

Count data regression

The Poisson process

$$P(y_i) = e^{-\lambda i}\lambda^{yi}/y_i!$$

This gives the probability of observing a count of y_i events, during a fixed interval. In order to condition the outcome (y) on a set of regressors (x), it is usually assumed that:

$$\lambda_i = E(y_i|x_i) = \exp(x_i\beta).$$

An important feature of the Poisson model is the equidispersion property, that $E(y_i|x_i) = Var(y_i|x_i) = \lambda_i$.

Maximum likelihood estimation (MLE) uses the fully specified probability distribution and maximises the log-likelihood:

$$LogL = \Sigma_i \log[P(y_i)]$$

The first-order moment condition implies an alternative formulation of the Poisson model, as a nonlinear regression equation:

$$E(y_i|x_i) = \exp(x_i\beta).$$

Overdispersion and the negbin model

The negative binomial specification allows for overdispersion by specifying, $\exp(x_i\beta + \mu_i) = [\exp(x_i\beta)]\eta_i$ where η_i is a gamma distributed error term. Then:

$$P(y_i) = \{\Gamma(y_i + \Psi_i)/\Gamma(\Psi_i)\Gamma(y_i + 1)\}(\Psi_i/(\lambda_i + \Psi_i))^{\Psi i}(\lambda_i/(\lambda_i + \Psi_i))^{yi},$$

where $\Gamma(.)$ is the gamma function. Letting the 'precision parameter' $\Psi = (1/a)\lambda^k$, for $a > 0$, gives:

$$E(y) = \lambda \text{ and } Var(y) = \lambda + a\lambda^{2-k}.$$

This leads to two special cases: setting $k = 1$ gives the negbin 1 model with the variance proportional to the mean, $(1 + a)\lambda$; and setting $k = 0$ gives the negbin 2 model where the variance is a quadratic function of the mean, $\lambda + a\lambda^2$. Setting $a = 0$ gives the Poisson model, and this nesting can be tested using a conventional t-test.

The 'zero inflated' or 'with zeros' model

The probability function for the zero inflated Poisson model, $P^{ZIP}(y|x)$ is related to the standard Poisson model, $P^P(y|x)$, as follows:

$$P^{ZIP}(y|x) = 1(y = 0)q + (1 - q)P^P(y|x).$$

Hurdle/two-part specifications

The hurdle model assumes the participation decision and the positive count are generated by separate probability processes $P_1(.)$ and $P_2(.)$. The log-likelihood for the hurdle model is:

$$LogL = \Sigma_{y=0} \log[1 - P_1(y > 0|x)] + \Sigma_{y>0} \{\log[P_1(y > 0|x)] + \log[P_2(y|x,y > 0)]\}$$

$$= \{\Sigma_{y=0} \log[1 - P_1(y > 0|x)] + \Sigma_{y>0} \log[P_1(y > 0|x)]\} + \{\Sigma_{y>0} \log[P_2(y|x,y > 0)]\}$$

$$= LogL_1 + LogL_2.$$

This shows that the two parts of the model can be estimated separately; with a binary process ($LogL_1$) and the truncated at zero count model ($LogL_2$).

The mixture approach

The mixture model or latent class model assumes that heterogeneity can be modelled using latent classes, where the probability of belonging to each class, j, is represented by a probability mass point, p_j. The C-point finite mixture negbin model takes the form:

$$P(y_i|.) = \Sigma^C_{j=1} p_j.P_j(y_i|.), \ \Sigma^C_{j=1} p_j = 1, \ 0 \leq p_j \leq 1,$$

where each of the $P_j(y_i|.)$ is a separate negbin model, and the p_js are estimated along with the other parameters of the model. This general form of the mixture model allows all of the parameters of the regression model (intercept and slopes) to vary across the classes. A special case is the finite density estimator, in which only the intercept varies. In this case the estimator can be interpreted as a discrete approximation of an underlying continuous distribution for the unobservable individual heterogeneity.

Duration analysis

Semiparametric models

In the Cox model, the hazard function at time t for individual i, $h_i(t, x_i)$, is defined as the product of a baseline hazard function, $h_o(t)$, and a proportionality factor $\exp(x_i\beta)$:

$$h_i(t, x_i) = h_o(t).exp(x_i \beta),$$

where x_i is a vector of covariates and β is a parameter vector.

Parametric models

Specifying the baseline hazard function as $h_o(t) = hpt^{p-1}$ gives the Weibull proportional hazards model:

$$h_i(t) = hpt^{p-1}.exp(x_i\beta),$$

where p is known as the shape parameter. The hazard is monotonically increasing for $p > 1$, showing increasing duration dependence, and monotonically decreasing for $p < 1$, showing decreasing duration dependence.

The hazard function, $h(t) = f(t)/S(t)$, can be used to derive the probability density function, $f(t)$, and the survival function, $S(t)$, for the Weibull model, and the likelihood function with right censoring is (using δ_i as an indicator of uncensored observations):

$$L = \Pi_i \{f_i(t)/S_i(t)\}^{\delta_i}.S_i(t).$$

Unobservable heterogeneity

Unobservable heterogeneity can be incorporated by adding a general heterogeneity effect μ and specifying:

$$f(t) = \int f(t|\mu)p(\mu)d\mu.$$

The unknown distribution $p(\mu)$ can be modelled parametrically using mixture distributions. Alternatively a non-parametric approach can be adopted which gives μ a discrete distribution characterised by the mass-points:

$$P(\mu = \mu_i) = p_i, I = 1, \dots , I,$$

where the parameters $(\mu_1, \dots , \mu_n, p_1, \dots , p_n)$ are estimated as part of the maximum likelihood estimation. This is the basis for the finite support density estimator.

Longitudinal data

Individual effects in panel data

To understand the role of individual effects in panel data models, consider the standard linear panel data regression model, in which there are repeated measurements $(t = 1, \dots , T)$ for a sample of n individuals $(I = 1, \dots , n)$:

$$y_{it} = x_{it}\beta + u_{it} = x_{it}\beta + \alpha_i + \varepsilon_{it}.$$

The presence of α_i implies clustering within individuals so that a random effects specification can improve the efficiency of the estimates of β. This stems from the structure imposed on the variance-covariance matrix of the error term:

$$\text{Var}[u_{it}] = E[u_{it}u_{is}] = \sigma_\alpha^2 + \sigma_\varepsilon^2, \ t = s$$

$$E[u_{it}u_{is}] = \sigma_\alpha^2, \ t \neq s.$$

These efficiency gains can be exploited to construct a generalised least squares (GLS) estimator.

Binary choices

Now consider a nonlinear model, for example the binary choice model:

$$P(y_{it} = 1) = P(\varepsilon_{it} > -x_{it}\beta - \alpha_i) = F(x_{it}\beta + \alpha_i).$$

This illustrates the so-called problem of incidental parameters. As $n \to \infty$, the number of parameters to be estimated (β, α_i) also grows. In linear models the estimators $\hat{\beta}$ and $\hat{\alpha}$ are asymptotically independent, which means that taking mean deviations or differencing the data allows the derivation of estimators for β whose limits do not depend on $\hat{\alpha}$. In general, this is not possible in nonlinear models and the inconsistency of estimates of α carries over into the estimates of β.

Random effects probit model

Assuming that α and ε are normally distributed and independent of x gives the random effects probit model (REP). In this case α can be integrated out to give the sample log-likelihood function:

$$\ln L = \sum_{i=1}^{n} \left\{ \ln \int_{-\infty}^{+\infty} \prod_{t=1}^{T} (\Phi[d_{it}(x_{it}\beta + \alpha)] \,)f(\alpha)d\alpha \right\},$$

where $d_{it} = 2y_{it} - 1$. This expression contains a univariate integral, which can be approximated by Gauss-Hermite quadrature. Assuming $\alpha \sim N(0, \sigma_\alpha^2)$, the contribution of each individual to the sample likelihood function is:

$$L_i = \int_{-\infty}^{+\infty} (1/\sqrt{2\pi\sigma_\alpha^2}) \exp(-\alpha^2/2\sigma_\alpha^2) \{ g(\alpha) \} d\alpha,$$

where

$$g(\alpha) = \prod_{t=1}^{T} \Phi[d_{it}(x_{it}\beta + \alpha)].$$

Use the change of variables, $\alpha = (\sqrt{2\sigma_\alpha^2})z$, to give:

$$L_i = (1/\sqrt{\pi}) \int_{-\infty}^{+\infty} \exp(-z^2) \{ g((\sqrt{2\sigma_\alpha^2})z) \} dz.$$

As it takes the generic form $\int_{-\infty}^{+\infty} \exp(-z^2)(f(z))dz$, this expression is suitable for Gauss-Hermite quadrature and can be approximated as a weighted sum:

$$L_i \approx (1/\sqrt{\pi}) \sum_{j=1}^{m} w_j \, g((\sqrt{2\sigma^2})a_j).$$

The finite mixture model

Deb (2001) applies a random effects probit model in which the distribution of the individual effect is approximated by a discrete density. In this case the sample log-likelihood is approximated by:

$$\ln L = \sum_{i=1}^{n} \ln \left(\sum_{j=1}^{C} \pi_j \left\{ \prod_{t=1}^{T} \Phi \left[d_{it}(x_{it}\beta + \alpha_j) \right] \right\} \right), \, 0 \leq \pi_j \leq 1, \sum_{j=1}^{C} \pi_j = 1.$$

Monte Carlo experiments show that only 3–4 points of support are required for the discrete density to mimic normal and chi-square densities sufficiently well so as to provide approximately unbiased estimates of the structural parameters and the variance of the individual effect.

The conditional logit estimator

The conditional logit estimator uses the fact that $\Sigma_t y_{it}$ is a sufficient statistic for α_i. This means that conditioning on $\Sigma_t y_{it}$ allows a consistent estimator for β to be derived. Using the logistic function:

$$P(y_{it} = 1) = F(X'_{it}\beta + \alpha_i) = \exp(x_{it}\beta + \alpha_i)/(1 + \exp(x_{it}\beta + \alpha_i)).$$

Concentrating on the case where $t = 2$, it is possible to show that:

$$P[(0,1)|(0,1) \text{ or } (1,0)] = \exp((x_{i2} - x_{i1})\beta)/(1 + \exp((x_{i2} - x_{i1})'\beta)).$$

This implies that a standard logit model can be applied to differenced data and the individual effect is swept out. In practice, conditioning on those observations that make a transition – (0,1) or (1,0) – and discarding those that do not – (0,0) or (1,1) – means that identification of the models relies on those observations where the dependent variable changes over time.

Parameterising the individual effect

Another approach to dealing with individual effects that are correlated with the regressors is to specify $E(\alpha|x)$ directly. For example:

$$\alpha_i = x_i\alpha + u_i, \, u_i \sim \text{iid } N(0, \sigma^2),$$

where $x_i = (x_{i1}, \dots, x_{iT})$, the values of the regressors for every wave of the panel, and $\alpha = (\alpha_1, \dots, \alpha_T)$. Then, by substituting, the distribution of y_{it} conditional on x but marginal to α_i has the probit form:

$$P(y_{it} = 1) = \Phi[(1 + \sigma^2)^{-\frac{1}{2}}(x_{it}\beta + x_i\alpha)].$$

The model could be estimated as a random effects probit to retrieve the parameters of interest (β, σ). This approach can also be applied in a random effects probit model with state dependence. In this case the initial values of the dependent variable are also included in order to deal with the problem that the initial conditions are correlated with the individual effect (the so-called 'initial conditions' problem).

Software appendix: full Stata code

This is the program to estimate the models described in this book using Stata. The code is written in a general format with the dependent variables called yvar (created using 'gen yvar = ...') and the list of independent variables called $xvars (created using 'global xvars 'male age... ."). The estimation sample for each model can be selected using the 'if' command, e.g. observations from the first wave of HALS can be selected by 'if wave==1'.

```
STATA PROGRAM FOR ANALYSIS OF THE HEALTH AND LIFESTYLE SURVEY
/* CHAPTER 2: SIMPLE DESCRIPTIVE STATISTICS */

/* LOAD THE STATA DATASET */
use 'c:\....\...\your_filename.dta', clear

/* CREATE A LOG FILE TO SAVE THE OUTPUT */
log using 'c:\...\...\your_filename.log', replace

/* CREATE GLOBAL FOR LIST OF VARIABLES TO BE USED IN MODELS */
global xvars 'male age age2 age3 ethbawi ethipb ethothnw
part unemp retd stdnt keephse
lsch14u lsch14 lsch15 lsch17 lsch18 lsch19
regsc1s regsc2 regsc3n regsc4 regsc5n
widow single seprd divorce
partime retired student keephouse'

/* DESCRIPTIVE STATISTICS */
summ $xvars

/* SOME DESCRIPTIVE ANALYSIS OF NON-RESPONSE */
gen yvar = sah
quietly regr yvar $xvars
gen miss=0
recode miss 0=1 if e(sample)
sort miss
by miss: summ $xvars


/* CHAPTER 3: BINARY CHOICES */

/* SELF-ASSESSED HEALTH */

* LINEAR PROBABILITY MODEL (OLS & WLS)

regress yvar $xvars, robust
predict yf

* SAVE COEFFICIENTS
matrix blpm=e(b)
matrix list blpm
scalar bun_lpm=_b[unemp]
scalar list bun_lpm

* WEIGHTED LEAST SQUARES
gen wt=1/(yf*(1-yf))
regress yvar $xvars [aweight=wt]
```

```
* RESET TEST
gen yf2=yf^2
quietly regress yvar $xvars yf2, robust
test yf2=0

drop wt yf yf2
* PROBIT MODEL
probit yvar $xvars
predict yf, xb

* PARTIAL EFFECTS (AT MEANS)
dprobit yvar $xvars

* SAVE COEFFICIENTS
matrix bpbt=e(b)
matrix list bpbt
scalar bun_pbt=_b[unemp]
scalar bun_pbt18=_b[unemp]*1.8
scalar bun_pbt16=_b[unemp]*1.6
scalar list bun_pbt bun_pbt18 bun_pbt16

scalar bm_pbt=_b[male]
gen mepbt_male = bm_pbt*normden(yf)

* MARGINAL EFFECTS
gen mepbt_unemp=bun_pbt*normden(yf)

* AVERAGE EFFECTS
gen aepbt_unemp=0
replace aepbt_unemp=norm(yf+bun_pbt)-norm(yf) if unemp==0
replace aepbt_unemp=norm(yf)-norm(yf-bun_pbt) if unemp==1
summ mepbt_unemp aepbt_unemp

* RESET TEST
gen yf2=yf^2
quietly probit yvar $xvars yf2
test yf2=0

drop yf yf2

* LOGIT MODEL
logit yvar $xvars
mfx compute if e(sample)
predict yf, xb

* SAVE COEFFICIENTS
matrix blgt=e(b)
matrix list blgt
scalar bun_lgt=_b[unemp]
scalar list bun_lgt bun_pbt18 bun_pbt16

* MARGINAL EFFECTS
gen melgt_unemp=bun_lgt*( exp(yf)/(1+exp(yf)))*(1-
exp(yf)/(1+exp(yf)))
* AVERAGE EFFECTS
gen aelgt_unemp=0
replace aelgt_unemp=exp(yf+bun_lgt)/(1+exp(yf+bun_lgt))-
exp(yf)/(1+exp(yf)) if unemp==0
```

```
replace aelgt_unemp=exp(yf)/(1+exp(yf))-exp(yf-bun_lgt)/
(1+exp(yf-bun_lgt)) if unemp==1
summ mepbt_unemp aepbt_unemp melgt_unemp aelgt_unemp
scalar list bun_lpm

* RESET TEST
gen yf2=yf^2
quietly logit yvar $xvars yf2
test yf2=0
drop yf yf2

/* CHAPTER 4: ORDERED PROBIT MODEL */

replace yvar=saho

oprobit yvar $xvars, table
predict yhat
predict yf, xb
gen yf2=yf^2

* PARTIAL EFFECTS FOR P(Y=0)

mfx compute, predict(outcome(0))

scalar mu1=_b[_cut1]
scalar bunemp=_b[unemp]
gen aeop_unemp=0
replace aeop_unemp=norm(mu1-yf-bunemp)-norm(mu1-yf) if unemp==0
replace aeop_unemp=norm(mu1-yf)-norm(mu1-yf+bunemp) if unemp==1
summ aeop_unemp
hist aeop_unemp

* RESET test
quietly oprobit yvar $xvars yf2
test yf2=0
drop yf yf2

/* CHAPTER 5: MULTINOMIAL LOGIT MODEL */

* FOR HEALTH CARE USE

gen hosp=hospop==1 | hospip==1
tab visitgp hosp
gen use = 0
replace use=1 if visitgp==1 & hosp==0
replace use=2 if hosp==1
replace use=. if visitgp==.
tab use

* MULTINOMIAL LOGIT
replace yvar=use
mlogit yvar $xvars

* Hausman test of IIA
est store hall
mlogit yvar $zvars if yvar!=2
est store hpartial
hausman hpartial hall, alleqs constant
```

```
/* CHAPTER 6: BIVARIATE PROBIT MODEL */

gen yvar1=regfag
gen yvar2=sah

biprobit yvar1 yvar2 $xvars
predict yf1, xb1
predict yf2, xb2
drop yf1 yf2

* PARTIAL EFFECT ON MARGINAL DISTRIBUTION
scalar bun_pbt=_b[yvar:unemp]
gen aepbt_unemp=0
replace aepbt_unemp=norm(yf1+bun_pbt)-norm(yf1) if unemp==0
replace aepbt_unemp=norm(yf1)-norm(yf1-bun_pbt) if unemp==1
summ aepbt_unemp
hist aepbt_unemp


/* CHAPTER 7: SELECTION BIAS */

* Sample Selection models (SSM) (Heckman selection
model/Generalised Tobit model)
* Heckman maximum likelihood estimates (FIML)
heckman lncig $xvars, select($xvars)
* Heckman two step consistent estimates
heckman lncig $xvars, select($xvars) twostep mills(imr)¨

probit regfag $xvars
predict yfp, xb
regre imr $quaneq
twoway scatter imr yfp


/* CHAPTER 8: THE EVALUATION PROBLEM */

* LINEAR OUTCOME (y2) BINARY TREATMENT (y1)

* THE EVALUATION PROBLEM

replace yvar2=hyfev1
replace yvar1=regfag

* "SELECTION ON OBSERVABLES" APPROACHES:-

* i. STANDARD PROBIT MODEL

regress yvar2 yvar1 $xvars
* ii. INVERSE PROBABILITY WEIGHTED ESTIMATOR

probit yvar1 $xvars
predict pi, p
gen ipw = 1
replace ipw =1/pi if yvar1 == 1
replace ipw=1/(1-pi) if yvar2 == 0
summ ipw

regress yvar2 yvar1 [pweight=ipw]

* iii. PROPENSITY SCORE MATCHING (DEFAULT OPTION)

psmatch2 yvar1 $xvars, out(yvar2)
```

```
* 'SELECTION ON UNOBSERVABLES' APPROACHES:

* HECKMAN TREATMENT EFFECTS MODEL

regr yvar2 yvar1 $zvars
treatreg yvar2 $xvars, treat(yvar1 = $zvars) twostep
treatreg yvar2 $xvars, treat(yvar1 = $zvars)

* INSTRUMENTAL VARIABLES ESTIMATOR

ivreg yvar2 $xvars (yvar1 = $zvars)
* BINARY OUTCOME (y2) BINARY TREATMENT (y1)

*RECURSIVE BIVARIATE PROBIT MODEL
probit yvar2 yvar1 $xvars
dprobit yvar2 yvar1 $xvars

biprobit (yvar2=yvar1 $xvars) (yvar1=$xvars)
predict yf1, xb1
predict yf2, xb2

* AVERAGE TREATMENT EFFECT (ATE)
scalar b1_pbt=_b[yvar1]
scalar rho=_b[athrho:_cons]
gen ate=0
replace ate=norm(yf1+b1_pbt)-norm(yf1) if yvar1==0
replace ate=norm(yf1)-norm(yf1-b1_pbt) if yvar1==1
summ ate
hist ate

* AVERAGE TREATMENT EFFECT ON THE TREATED (ATET)
gen atet=0
replace atet=norm((yf1+b1_pbt-rho*yf2)/(1-rho^2)^0.5)-norm((yf1-
rho*yf2)/(1-rho^2)^0.5) if yvar1==0
replace atet= norm((yf1-rho*yf2)/(1-rho^2)^0.5)-norm((yf1-b1_pbt-
rho*yf2)/(1-rho^2)^0.5) if yvar1==1
summ atet if yvar1==1
hist atet if yvar1==1

drop yf1 yf2 ate atet


/* CHAPTER 9: COUNT DATA REGRESSSIONS */

replace yvar=fagday

* POISSON REGRESSION
poisson yvar $xvars
* predict exp(xb)
predict fitted, n
predict yf, xb
gen yf2=yf^2

*PARTIAL EFFECTS
scalar bunemp=_b[unemp]
gen ae_unemp=0
replace ae_unemp=exp(yf+bunemp)-exp(yf) if unemp==0
replace ae_unemp=exp(yf)-exp(yf-bunemp) if unemp==1
summ ae_unemp
hist ae_unemp
```

```
scalar drop bunemp
drop ae_unemp

* TABULATE ACTUAL AND FITTED VALUES OF Y

replace fitted=round(fitted)
tab yvar
tab fitted
tab fitted yvar

* RESET TEST
quietly poisson yvar $xvars yf2
test yf2

* Pseudo-ML-robust standard errors
poisson yvar $xvars, robust

drop fitted yf

* NEGBIN REGRESSION (NEGBIN2)
nbreg yvar $xvars

predict yf, xb
predict fitted

*PARTIAL EFFECTS
scalar bunemp=_b[unemp]
gen ae_unemp=0
replace ae_unemp=exp(yf+bunemp)-exp(yf) if unemp==0
replace ae_unemp=exp(yf)-exp(yf-bunemp) if unemp==1
summ ae_unemp
hist ae_unemp
scalar drop bunemp
drop ae_unemp

replace fitted=round(fitted)
tab fitted yvar
drop fitted

* GENERALISED NEGBIN ln(a)=zd
set matsize 100
gnbreg yvar $xvars, lna($xvars)

predict fitted
replace fitted=round(fitted)
tab fitted yvar
drop fitted

* ZERO-INFLATED POISSON AND NEGBIN MODELS
zip yvar $xvars, inflate(_cons) vuong
predict fitted
predict yf
replace fitted=round(fitted)
tab fitted yvar
drop fitted

*PARTIAL EFFECTS FOR ZIP
scalar bunemp=_b[unemp]
scalar qi=_b[inflate:_cons]
```

```
scalar qi=exp(qi)/(1+exp(qi))
scalar list qi
gen ae_unemp=0
replace ae_unemp=(1-qi)*(exp(yf+bunemp)-exp(yf)) if unemp==0
replace ae_unemp=(1-qi)*(exp(yf)-exp(yf-bunemp)) if unemp==1
summ ae_unemp
hist ae_unemp
scalar drop bunemp
drop ae_unemp

zip yvar $xvars, inflate($xvars _cons)

predict pi, p
predict fitted

replace fitted=round(fitted)
tab fitted yvar
drop fitted

/*zinb yvar $xvars, inflate(_cons) vuong
predict fitted
replace fitted=round(fitted)
tab fitted yvar
drop fitted

zinb yvar $xvars, inflate($xvars|_cons) vuong
predict fitted
replace fitted=round(fitted)
tab fitted yvar
drop fitted*/

drop pi

* HURDLE MODELS
replace yvar1=regfag
logit yvar1 $xvars
predict yf1, xb
predict pi, p

ztp yvar $xvars
ztnb yvar $xvars


/* CHAPTER 10: DURATION ANALYSIS */

/*SURVIVAL TIME is LIFESPAN if the ENTRY DATE is the DATE OF
BIRTH and the EXIT DATE is June 2005*/
/*LIFESPAN is LEFT TRUNCATED: DURATION IS OBSERVED ONLY FOR THOSE
WHO SURVIVED UP TO THE INTERVIEW DATE*/

stset lifespan, failure(death) id(serno) time0(age)

stsum
stdes

/***PLOT HAZARD AND SURVIVAL FUNCTIONS***/
sts graph, na title('NA ls') saving(lsNA, replace)
sts graph, hazard  title('KM hazard ls') saving(lsHkm, replace)
sts graph, title('KM Survival ls') saving(lsKMsurv, replace)
```

```
/* Cox PH model */
stcox $xls

/*** WEIBULL MODEL***/
streg $xls, d(weibull) nolog /*PH version */
streg $xls, d(weibull) nolog time /*AFT Version*/
stcurve, survival title('Ls survival') saving(lssurv, replace)
stcurve, cumh title('Ls cumh') saving(lscumh, replace)
stcurve, hazard title('Ls hazard') saving(lshaz, replace)

/* CHAPTER 11: PANEL DATA */

* SET INDIVIDUAL (i) AND TIME (t) INDEXES
iis serno
tis wave
sort serno wave

/* THE FOLLOWING COMMANDS CREATE INDICATORS OF WHETHER
OBSERVATIONS ARE IN THE BALANCED AND UNBALANCED ESTIMATION SAM-
PLES */

Replace yvar=fagday

quietly regr yvar $xvars, robust cluster(pid)
gen insampm = 0
recode insampm 0 = 1 if e(sample)
sort serno wave
gen constant = 1
by serno: egen Ti = sum(constant) if insampm == 1
drop constant
sort wave
by serno: gen nextwavem = insampm[_n+1]
gen allwavesm = .
recode allwavesm . = 0 if Ti ~= 8
recode allwavesm . = 1 if Ti == 8
gen numwavesm = .
replace numwavesm = Ti

* LIST OF Xit PLUS MUNDLAK SPECIFICATION
by serno: egen munemp=mean(unemp)
etc...

global xvarsm '...'

/* LINEAR PANEL DATA MODELS */

* SUMMARY STATISTICS - UNBALANCED SAMPLE
xtsum yvar $xvars

* POOLED REGRESSION - UNBALANCED SAMPLE
regr yvar $xvars

* WITH ROBUST & CLUSTER TO ALLOW FOR REPEATED OBSERVATIONS
regr yvar $xvars, robust cluster(serno)

* MUNDLAK WITH ROBUST & CLUSTER TO ALLOW FOR REPEATED
OBSERVATIONS
regr yvar $xvarsm, robust cluster(serno)
```

```
* PANEL DATA REGRESSIONS-UNBALANCED SAMPLE

* RANDOM EFFECTS MODEL (RE)
xtreg yvar $xvars, re
* LM TEST FOR SIGNIFICANCE OF INDIVIDUAL EFFECTS
xttest0
* HAUSMAN TEST FOR RE V. FE COEFFICIENTS
xthaus

* RANDOM EFFECTS MODEL (RE)
xtreg yvar $xvars if allwavesm==1, re
* LM TEST FOR SIGNIFICANCE OF INDIVIDUAL EFFECTS
xttest0
* HAUSMAN TEST FOR RE V. FE COEFFICIENTS
xthaus

* RANDOM EFFECTS MODEL (RE) WITH MUNDLAK ($XVARSM)
xtreg yvar $xvarsm, re
xthaus
xtreg yvar $xvarsm if allwavesm==1, re
xthaus

* LEAST SQUARES DUMMY VARIABLE REGRESSION (LSDV)

global zvars 'male etc …'

areg yvar $xvars, absorb(serno)
predict ai, d
regress ai $zvars if wavenum==1

* FIXED EFFECTS MODEL (FE)
xtreg yvar $xvars, fe
xtreg yvar $xvars if allwavesm==1, fe

* BETWEEN EFFECTS MODEL (BE)
xtreg yvar $xvars, be


/* NONLINEAR PANEL DATA MODELS */

replace yvar=sah

* SUMMARY STATISTICS
xtsum yvar $xvars
xtsum yvar $xvars if allwavesm==1

* POOLED PROBIT-DPROBIT USED TO OBTAIN APEs
dprobit yvar $xvars
dprobit yvar $xvars if allwavesm==1
* USING ROBUST INFERENCE TO ALLOW FOR CLUSTERING WITHIN 'I'
dprobit yvar $xvars, robust cluster(serno)
dprobit yvar $xvars if allwavesm==1, robust cluster(serno)

* PANEL RE PROBIT
xtprobit yvar $xvars
quadchk
xtprobit yvar $xvars if allwavesm==1
quadchk
```

```
* RANDOM EFFECTS MODEL (RE) WITH MUNDLAK
xtprobit yvar $xvarsm
quadchk
xtprobit yvar $xvarsm if allwavesm==1
quadchk

* CONDITIONAL ("FIXED EFFECTS") LOGIT MODEL (FE)
clogit yvar $xvars, group(serno)
clogit yvar $xvars if allwavesm==1, group(serno)
```

References

Auld MC. Using observational data to identify causal effects of health-related behaviour. In: Jones AM, editor. *Elgar Companion to Health Economics*. Edward Elgar; 2006.

Blundell RW, Smith RJ. Simultaneous microeconometric models with censored or qualitative dependent variables. In: Maddala GS, Rao CR, Vinod HD, editors. *Handbook of Statistics*, vol. 11. Elsevier; 1993.

Cox BD *et al. The Health and Lifestyle Survey*. The Health Promotion Research Trust; 1987.

Cox BD, Huppert FA, Whichelow MJ. *The Health and Lifestyle Survey: seven years on*. Aldershot: Dartmouth; 1993.

Deb P. A discrete random effects probit model with application to the demand for preventive care. *Health Econ*. 2001; **10**: 371–83.

Deb P, Trivedi PK. Demand for medical care by the elderly: a finite mixture approach. *J Appl Econometrics*. 1997; **12**: 313–36.

Fitzgerald J, Gottshalk P, Moffitt R. An analysis of sample attrition in panel data. The Michigan Panel Study on Income Dynamics. *J Human Res*. 1998; **33**: 251–99.

Forster M, Jones AM. The role of taxes in starting and quitting smoking: duration analysis of British data. *J Roy Stat Soc (Series A)*. 2001; **164**: 517–47.

Heckman JJ. Sample selection bias as a specification error. *Econometrica* 1979; **47**: 153–61.

Jones AM. Health econometrics. In: Culyer AJ, Newhouse JP, editors. *Handbook of Health Economics*. Elsevier; 2000.

Manning W. Dealing with skewed data on costs and expenditures. In: Jones AM, editor. *Elgar Companion to Health Economics*. Edward Elgar; 2006.

Mullahy J. Heterogeneity, excess zeros, and the structure of count data models. *J Appl Econometrics*. 1997; **12**: 337–50.

Train KE. *Discrete Choice Methods with Simulation*. Cambridge University Press; 2003.

Index